This report contains the collective ... arily represent the decisions
or the stated policy of the W ... ation of the United Nations

Report Series
916

DIET, NUTRITION AND THE PREVENTION OF CHRONIC DISEASES

Report of a
Joint WHO/FAO Expert Consultation

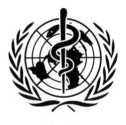

World Health Organization

Geneva 2003

WHO Library Cataloguing-in-Publication Data

Joint WHO/FAO Expert Consultation on Diet, Nutrition and the Prevention of
   Chronic Diseases (2002 : Geneva, Switzerland)
   Diet, nutrition and the prevention of chronic diseases: report of a joint WHO/FAO expert
   consultation, Geneva, 28 January – 1 February 2002.

   (WHO technical report series ; 916)

   1.Chronic disease – epidemiology 2.Diet – standards
   3.Feeding behavior 4.Energy metabolism 5.Motor activity
   6.Cost of illness I.Title II.Series.

   ISBN 92 4 120916 X   (NLM classification: QU 145)
   ISSN 0512-3054

Typeset and printed in Switzerland

Contents

Joint WHO/FAO Expert Consultation on Diet, Nutrition and the Prevention of Chronic Diseases

Geneva, 28 January–1 February 2002

Members

Dr E.K. Amine, Dean, High Institute of Public Health, Alexandria University, Alexandria, Egypt

Dr N.H. Baba, Chairperson, Department of Nutrition and Food Sciences, American University of Beirut, Beirut, Lebanon

Dr M. Belhadj, Professor of Internal Medicine and Diabetologia, Centre Hospitalier Universitaire, Oran, Algeria

Dr M. Deurenberg-Yap, Director, Research and Information Management, Health Promotion Board, Singapore (*Co-Rapporteur*)

Dr A. Djazayery, Professor of Nutrition, Department of Nutrition and Biochemistry, School of Public Health, Tehran University of Medical Sciences, Tehran, Islamic Republic of Iran

Dr T. Forrester, Director, Tropical Medicine Research Institute, The University of the West Indies, Kingston, Jamaica

Dr D.A. Galuska, Division of Nutrition and Physical Activity, National Center for Chronic Disease, Prevention and Health Promotion, Centers for Disease Control and Prevention, Atlanta, GA, USA

Dr S. Herman, Senior Researcher, Nutrition Research and Development Centre, Ministry of Health, Bogor, Indonesia

Professor W.P.T. James, Chairman, International Obesity Task Force, London, England

Dr J.R. M'Buyamba Kabangu, Hypertension Unit, Department of Internal Medicine, University of Kinshasa Hospital, Kinshasa, Democratic Republic of the Congo

Professor M.B. Katan, Division of Human Nutrition and Epidemiology, Wageningen University, Wageningen, Netherlands

Dr T.J. Key, Cancer Research UK, Epidemiology Unit, University of Oxford, The Radcliffe Infirmary, Oxford, England

Professor S. Kumanyika, Center for Clinical Epidemiology and Biostatistics, School of Medicine, University of Pennsylvania, Philadelphia, PA, USA (*Vice-Chairperson*)

Professor J. Mann, Department of Human Nutrition, University of Otago, Dunedin, New Zealand

Dr P.J. Moynihan, School of Dental Sciences, University of Newcastle-upon-Tyne, Newcastle-upon-Tyne, England

Dr A.O. Musaiger, Director, Environmental and Biological Programme, Bahrain Centre for Studies and Research, Manama, Bahrain

Dr G.W. Olwit, Kampala, Uganda

Dr J. Petkeviciene, Institute for Biomedical Research, Kaunas Medical University, Kaunas, Lithuania

Dr A. Prentice, Director, Human Nutrition Research, Medical Research Council, Cambridge, England

Professor K.S. Reddy, Department of Cardiology, Cardiothoracic Centre, All India Institute of Medical Science, New Delhi, India

Dr A. Schatzkin, Nutritional Epidemiology Branch, National Cancer Institute, National Institute of Health, Rockville, MD, USA

Professor J.C. Seidell, National Institute of Public Health and the Environment, Bilthoven, Netherlands (*Co-Rapporteur*)

Dr A.P. Simopoulos, President, The Center for Genetics, Nutrition and Health, Washington, DC, USA

Professor S. Srianujata, Director, Institute of Nutrition, Mahidol University, Nakhon Pathom, Thailand

Dr N. Steyn, Chronic Diseases of Lifestyle, Medical Research Council, Tygerberg, South Africa

Professor B. Swinburn, School of Health Sciences, Deakin University, Melbourne, Victoria, Australia

Dr R. Uauy, Institute of Nutrition and Food Technology, University of Chile, Santiago, Chile; and Department of Epidemiology and Population Health, London School of Hygiene and Tropical Medicine, London, England (*Chairperson*)

Dr M. Wahlqvist, Director, Asia Pacific Health and Nutrition Centre, Monash Asia Institute, Monash University, Melbourne, Victoria, Australia

Professor Wu Zhao-Su, Institute of Heart, Lung and Blood Vessel Diseases, Beijing, China

Dr N. Yoshiike, Division of Health and Nutrition Monitoring, National Institute of Health and Nutrition, Tokyo, Japan

Representatives of other organizations[*]

United Nations Administrative Committee on Coordination/Subcommittee on Nutrition (ACC/SCN),

Dr S. Rabenek, Technical Secretary, ACC/SCN, Geneva, Switzerland

Secretariat[†]

Dr K. Bagchi, Regional Adviser, Nutrition, Food Security and Safety, WHO Regional Office for the Eastern Mediterranean, Cairo, Egypt

Dr T. Cavalli-Sforza, Regional Adviser, Nutrition, WHO Regional Office for the Western Pacific, Manila, Philippines

---

[*] Unable to attend: International Atomic Energy Agency, Vienna, Austria; Secretariat of the Pacific Community, Noumea, New Caledonia; United Nations Children's Fund, New York, NY, USA; United Nations University, Tokyo, Japan; World Bank, Washington, DC, USA.

[†] Unable to attend: Dr H. Delgado, Director, Institute of Nutrition of Central America and Panama, Guatemala City, Guatemala; Dr F.J. Henry, Director, Caribbean Food and Nutrition Institute, The University of the West Indies, Kingston, Jamaica.

Dr G.A. Clugston, Director, Department of Nutrition for Health and Development, Sustainable Development and Healthy Environments, WHO, Geneva, Switzerland

Dr I. Darnton-Hill, Department of Noncommunicable Disease Prevention and Health Promotion, Noncommunicable Diseases and Mental Health, WHO, Geneva, Switzerland

Professor A. Ferro-Luzzi, National Institute for Food and Nutrition Research, Rome, Italy (*Temporary Adviser*)

Dr J. Leowski, Regional Adviser, Noncommunicable Diseases, WHO Regional Office for South-East Asia, New Delhi, India

Dr C. Nishida, Department of Nutrition for Health and Development, Sustainable Development and Healthy Environments, WHO, Geneva, Switzerland (*Secretary*)

Dr D. Nyamwaya, Medical Officer, Health Promotion, WHO Regional Office for Africa, Harare, Zimbabwe

Dr A. Ouedraogo, Regional Officer, Nutrition, WHO Regional Office for Africa, Harare, Zimbabwe

Dr P. Pietinen, Department of Noncommunicable Disease Prevention and Health Promotion, Noncommunicable Diseases and Mental Health, WHO, Geneva, Switzerland

Dr P. Puska, Director, Department of Noncommunicable Disease Prevention and Health Promotion, Noncommunicable Diseases and Mental Health, WHO, Geneva, Switzerland

Dr E. Riboli, International Agency for Research on Cancer, Lyon, France

Dr A. Robertson, Regional Adviser, Nutrition and Food Security Programme, WHO Regional Office for Europe, Copenhagen, Denmark

Dr P. Shetty, Chief, Nutrition Planning, Assessment and Evaluation Service, Food and Nutrition Division, FAO, Rome, Italy

Dr R. Weisell, Nutrition Planning, Assessment and Evaluation Service, Food and Nutrition Division, FAO, Rome, Italy

Dr D. Yach, Executive Director, Noncommunicable Diseases and Mental Health, WHO, Geneva, Switzerland

Abbreviations

The following abbreviations are used in this report:

ACC	United Nations Administrative Committee on Coordination
AIDS	acquired immunodeficiency syndrome
BMI	body mass index
CARMEN	Carbohydrate Ratio Management in European National diets
CHD	coronary heart disease
CVD	cardiovascular disease
DALY	disability-adjusted life year
DASH	dietary approaches to stop hypertension
DEXA	dual-energy X-ray absorptiometry
DHA	docosahexaenoic acid
dmf	decayed, missing, filled primary (teeth)
DMF	decayed, missing, filled permanent (teeth)
dmft	decayed, missing, filled primary teeth
DMFT	decayed, missing, filled permanent teeth
DONALD	Dortmund Nutritional and Anthropometric Longitudinally Designed Study
ECC	early childhood caries
EPA	eicosapentaenoic acid
EPIC	European Prospective Investigation into Cancer and Nutrition
ERGOB	European Research Group for Oral Biology
FAOSTAT	Food and Agricultural Organization of the United Nations Statistical Databases
FER	fat to energy ratio
GDP	gross domestic product
GISSI	Gruppo Italiano por lo Studio della Sopravvivenza nell'Infarto Miocardico
GNP	gross national product
HBP	high blood pressure
HDL	high-density lipoprotein
HFI	hereditary fructose intolerance
HIV	human immunodeficiency virus
HOPE	Heart Outcomes Prevention Evaluation
IARC	International Agency for Research on Cancer
IDDM	insulin-dependent diabetes mellitus
IGT	impaired glucose tolerance
IHD	ischaemic heart disease

IUGR	intrauterine growth retardation
LDL	low-density lipoprotein
MGRS	multicentre growth reference study (i.e. the WHO MGRS study)
mRNA	messenger ribonucleic acid
MSG	monosodium glutamate
MUFA	monounsaturated fatty acid
NCD	noncommunicable disease
NGO	nongovernmental organization
NIDDM	non-insulin-dependent diabetes mellitus
NSP	non-starch polysaccharides
PUFA	polyunsaturated fatty acid
RCT	randomized controlled trial
SCN	ACC Subcommittee on Nutrition[1]
SFA	saturated fatty acid
T1DM	type 1 diabetes
T2DM	type 2 diabetes
VLDL	very low-density lipoprotein
WCRF	World Cancer Research Fund
WHR	waist:hip circumference ratio or waist:hip ratio

---

[1] In April 2002 the name of the Subcommittee on Nutrition was changed to the United Nations System Standing Committee on Nutrition.

1. Introduction

A Joint WHO/FAO Expert Consultation on Diet, Nutrition and the Prevention of Chronic Diseases met in Geneva from 28 January to 1 February 2002. The meeting was opened by Dr D. Yach, Executive Director, Noncommunicable Diseases and Mental Health, WHO, on behalf of the Directors-General of the Food and Agriculture Organization of the United Nations and the World Health Organization. The Consultation followed up the work of a WHO Study Group on Diet, Nutrition and Prevention of Noncommunicable Diseases, which had met in 1989 to make recommendations regarding the prevention of chronic diseases and the reduction of their impact (1). The Consultation recognized that the growing epidemic of chronic disease afflicting both developed and developing countries was related to dietary and lifestyle changes and undertook the task of reviewing the considerable scientific progress that has been made in different areas. For example, there is better epidemiological evidence for determining certain risk factors, and the results of a number of new controlled clinical trials are now available. The mechanisms of the chronic disease process are clearer, and interventions have been demonstrated to reduce risk.

During the past decade, rapid expansion in a number of relevant scientific fields and, in particular, in the amount of population-based epidemiological evidence has helped to clarify the role of diet in preventing and controlling morbidity and premature mortality resulting from noncommunicable diseases (NCDs). Some of the specific dietary components that increase the probability of occurrence of these diseases in individuals, and interventions to modify their impact, have also been identified.

Furthermore, rapid changes in diets and lifestyles that have occurred with industrialization, urbanization, economic development and market globalization, have accelerated over the past decade. This is having a significant impact on the health and nutritional status of populations, particularly in developing countries and in countries in transition. While standards of living have improved, food availability has expanded and become more diversified, and access to services has increased, there have also been significant negative consequences in terms of inappropriate dietary patterns, decreased physical activities and increased tobacco use, and a corresponding increase in diet-related chronic diseases, especially among poor people.

Food and food products have become commodities produced and traded in a market that has expanded from an essentially local base to an increasingly global one. Changes in the world food economy are reflected in shifting dietary patterns, for example, increased consumption of energy-dense diets high in fat, particularly saturated fat, and low in unrefined carbohydrates. These patterns are combined with a decline in energy expenditure that is associated with a sedentary lifestyle — motorized transport, labour-saving devices in the home, the phasing out of physically demanding manual tasks in the workplace, and leisure time that is preponderantly devoted to physically undemanding pastimes.

Because of these changes in dietary and lifestyle patterns, chronic NCDs — including obesity, diabetes mellitus, cardiovascular disease (CVD), hypertension and stroke, and some types of cancer — are becoming increasingly significant causes of disability and premature death in both developing and newly developed countries, placing additional burdens on already overtaxed national health budgets.

The Consultation provided an opportune moment for FAO and WHO to draw on the latest scientific evidence available and to update recommendations for action to governments, international agencies and concerned partners in the public and private sectors. The overall aim of these recommendations is to implement more effective and sustainable policies and strategies to deal with the increasing public health challenges related to diet and health.

The Consultation articulated a new platform, not just of dietary and nutrient targets, but of a concept of the human organism's subtle and complex relationship to its environment in relation to chronic diseases. The discussions took into account ecological, societal and behavioural aspects beyond causative mechanisms. The experts looked at diet within the context of the macroeconomic implications of public health recommendations on agriculture, and the global supply and demand for foodstuffs, both fresh and processed. The role of diet in defining the expression of genetic susceptibility to NCDs, the need for responsible and creative partnerships with both traditional and non-traditional partners, and the importance of addressing the whole life course, were all recognized.

Nutrition is coming to the fore as a major modifiable determinant of chronic disease, with scientific evidence increasingly supporting the view that alterations in diet have strong effects, both positive and negative, on health throughout life. Most importantly, dietary adjustments may not only influence present health, but may determine whether or not an individual will develop such diseases as cancer, cardiovascular disease and diabetes much later in life. However, these concepts have not led to a change in policies or in practice. In many developing countries, food policies remain focused only on undernutrition and are not addressing the prevention of chronic disease.

2

Although the primary purpose of the Consultation was to examine and develop recommendations for diet and nutrition in the prevention of chronic diseases, the need for sufficient physical activity was also discussed and is therefore emphasized in the report. This emphasis is consistent with the trend to consider physical activity alongside the complex of diet, nutrition and health. Some relevant aspects include:

- Energy expenditure through physical activity is an important part of the energy balance equation that determines body weight. A decrease in energy expenditure through decreased physical activity is likely to be one of the major factors contributing to the global epidemic of overweight and obesity.

- Physical activity has great influence on body composition — on the amount of fat, muscle and bone tissue.

- To a large extent, physical activity and nutrients share the same metabolic pathways and can interact in various ways that influence the risk and pathogenesis of several chronic diseases.

- Cardiovascular fitness and physical activity have been shown to reduce significantly the effects of overweight and obesity on health.

- Physical activity and food intake are both specific and mutually interacting behaviours that are and can be influenced partly by the same measures and policies.

- Lack of physical activity is already a global health hazard and is a prevalent and rapidly increasing problem in both developed and developing countries, particularly among poor people in large cities.

In order to achieve the best results in preventing chronic diseases, the strategies and policies that are applied must fully recognize the essential role of diet, nutrition and physical activity.

This report calls for a shift in the conceptual framework for developing strategies for action, placing nutrition — together with the other principal risk factors for chronic disease, namely, tobacco use and alcohol consumption — at the forefront of public health policies and programmes.

Reference

1. *Diet, nutrition, and the prevention of chronic diseases. Report of a WHO Study Group.* Geneva, World Health Organization, 1990 (WHO Technical Report Series, No. 797).

2. Background

2.1 The global burden of chronic diseases

Diet and nutrition are important factors in the promotion and maintenance of good health throughout the entire life course. Their role as determinants of chronic NCDs is well established and they therefore occupy a prominent position in prevention activities (1).

The latest scientific evidence on the nature and strength of the links between diet and chronic diseases is examined and discussed in detail in the following sections of this report. This section gives an overall view of the current situation and trends in chronic diseases at the global level. The chronic diseases considered in this report are those that are related to diet and nutrition and present the greatest public health burden, either in terms of direct cost to society and government, or in terms of disability-adjusted life years (DALYs). These include obesity, diabetes, cardio-vascular diseases, cancer, osteoporosis and dental diseases.

The burden of chronic diseases is rapidly increasing worldwide. It has been calculated that, in 2001, chronic diseases contributed approxi-mately 60% of the 56.5 million total reported deaths in the world and approximately 46% of the global burden of disease (1). The proportion of the burden of NCDs is expected to increase to 57% by 2020. Almost half of the total chronic disease deaths are attributable to cardiovascular diseases; obesity and diabetes are also showing worrying trends, not only because they already affect a large proportion of the population, but also because they have started to appear earlier in life.

The chronic disease problem is far from being limited to the developed regions of the world. Contrary to widely held beliefs, developing countries are increasingly suffering from high levels of public health problems related to chronic diseases. In five out of the six regions of WHO, deaths caused by chronic diseases dominate the mortality statistics (1). Although human immunodeficiency virus/acquired immunodeficiency syndrome (HIV/AIDS), malaria and tuberculosis, along with other infectious diseases, still predominate in sub-Saharan Africa and will do so for the foreseeable future, 79% of all deaths worldwide that are attributable to chronic diseases are already occurring in developing countries (2).

It is clear that the earlier labelling of chronic diseases as "diseases of affluence" is increasingly a misnomer, as they emerge both in poorer countries and in the poorer population groups in richer countries. This shift in the pattern of disease is taking place at an accelerating rate; furthermore, it is occurring at a faster rate in developing countries than it did in the industrialized regions of the world half a century ago (3). This rapid rate of change, together with the increasing burden of disease, is creating a major public health threat which demands immediate and effective action.

It has been projected that, by 2020, chronic diseases will account for almost three-quarters of all deaths worldwide, and that 71% of deaths due to ischaemic heart disease (IHD), 75% of deaths due to stroke, and 70% of deaths due to diabetes will occur in developing countries (4). The number of people in the developing world with diabetes will increase by more than 2.5-fold, from 84 million in 1995 to 228 million in 2025 (5). On a global basis, 60% of the burden of chronic diseases will occur in developing countries. Indeed, cardiovascular diseases are even now more numerous in India and China than in all the economically developed countries in the world put together (2). As for overweight and obesity, not only has the current prevalence already reached unprecedented levels, but the rate at which it is annually increasing in most developing regions is substantial (3). The public health implications of this phenomenon are staggering, and are already becoming apparent.

The rapidity of the changes in developing countries is such that a double burden of disease may often exist. India, for example, at present faces a combination of communicable diseases and chronic diseases, with the burden of chronic diseases just exceeding that of communicable diseases. Projections nevertheless indicate that communicable diseases will still occupy a critically important position up to 2020 (6). Another eloquent example is that of obesity, which is becoming a serious problem throughout Asia, Latin America and parts of Africa, despite the widespread presence of undernutrition. In some countries, the prevalence of obesity has doubled or tripled over the past decade.

Chronic diseases are largely preventable diseases. Although more basic research may be needed on some aspects of the mechanisms that link diet to health, the currently available scientific evidence provides a sufficiently strong and plausible basis to justify taking action now. Beyond the appropriate medical treatment for those already affected, the public health approach of primary prevention is considered to be the most cost-effective, affordable and sustainable course of action to cope with the chronic disease epidemic worldwide. The adoption of a common risk-factor approach to chronic disease prevention is a major development in the thinking behind an integrated health policy. Sometimes chronic diseases are considered communicable at the risk factor level (7). Modern dietary patterns and physical activity patterns are risk behaviours that travel across countries and are transferable from one population to another like an infectious disease, affecting disease patterns globally.

While age, sex and genetic susceptibility are non-modifiable, many of the risks associated with age and sex are modifiable. Such risks include behavioural factors (e.g. diet, physical inactivity, tobacco use, alcohol consumption); biological factors (e.g. dyslipidemia, hypertension, overweight, hyperinsulinaemia); and finally societal factors, which include a complex mixture of interacting socioeconomic, cultural and other environmental parameters.

Diet has been known for many years to play a key role as a risk factor for chronic diseases. What is apparent at the global level is that great changes have swept the entire world since the second half of the twentieth century, inducing major modifications in diet, first in industrial regions and more recently in developing countries. Traditional, largely plant-based diets have been swiftly replaced by high-fat, energy-dense diets with a substantial content of animal-based foods. But diet, while critical to prevention, is just one risk factor. Physical inactivity, now recognized as an increasingly important determinant of health, is the result of a progressive shift of lifestyle towards more sedentary patterns, in developing countries as much as in industrialized ones. Recent data from São Paulo, Brazil, for example, indicate that 70–80% of the population are remarkably inactive (8). The combination of these and other risk factors, such as tobacco use, is likely to have an additive or even a multiplier effect, capable of accelerating the pace at which the chronic disease epidemic is emerging in the developing countries.

The need for action to strengthen control and prevention measures to counter the spread of the chronic disease epidemic is now widely recognized by many countries, but the developing countries are lagging behind in implementing such measures. Encouragingly, however, efforts to counteract the rise in chronic diseases are increasingly being assigned a higher priority. This situation is reflected by the growing interest of Member States, the concerned international and bilateral agencies as well as nongovernmental organizations in addressing food and nutrition policy, health promotion, and strategy for the control and prevention of chronic diseases, as well as other related topics such as promoting healthy ageing and tobacco control. The 1992 International Conference on Nutrition specifically identified the need to prevent and control the increasing public health problems of chronic diseases by promoting appropriate diets and healthy lifestyles (9–11). The need to address chronic disease prevention from a broad-based perspective was also recognized by the World Health Assembly in 1998 (12) and again in 1999 (13). In 2000, the World Health Assembly passed a further resolution on the broad basis of the prevention and control of noncommunicable diseases (14), and in 2002 adopted a resolution that urged Member States to collaborate with WHO to develop "...a global strategy on diet, physical activity and health for the prevention and control of noncommunicable diseases, based on evidence and best practices, with special emphasis on an integrated approach..." (*15*).

Several factors have constrained progress in the prevention of chronic diseases. These include underestimation of the effectiveness of interventions, the belief of there being a long delay in achieving any measurable impact, commercial pressures, institutional inertia and inadequate resources. These aspects need to be taken seriously and combated. One example is provided by Finland. In North Karelia, age-adjusted mortality rates of coronary heart disease dropped dramatically between the early 1970s and 1995 (*16*). Analyses of the three main risk factors (smoking, high blood pressure, raised plasma cholesterol) indicate that diet — operating through lowering plasma cholesterol and blood pressure levels — accounted for the larger part of this substantial decline in cardiovascular disease. The contribution made by medication and treatment (antilipid and hypotensive drugs, surgery) was very small. Rather, the decline was largely achieved through community action and the pressure of consumer demand on the food market. The Finnish and other experience indicates that interventions can be effective, that dietary changes are important, that these changes can be strengthened by public demand, and finally that appreciable changes can take place very rapidly. The experience of the Republic of Korea is also notable since the community has largely maintained its traditional high-vegetable diet despite major social and economic change (*17*). The Republic of Korea has lower rates of chronic diseases and lower than expected level of fat intake and obesity prevalence than other industrialized countries with similar economic development (*18*).

There are several opportunities for new global and national actions, including strengthened interaction and partnerships; regulatory, legislative and fiscal approaches; and more stringent accountability mechanisms.

The broad parameters for a dialogue with the food industries are: less saturated fat; more fruits and vegetables; effective food labelling; and incentives for the marketing and production of healthier products. In working with advertising, media and entertainment partners, there is a need to stress the importance of clear and unambiguous messages to children and youths. Global "health and nutrition literacy" requires a vast increase in attention and resources.

Many studies show a relationship between health and income, with the poorest sections of the population being the most vulnerable. Poor people are at an increased social disadvantage in terms of the incidence of chronic diseases, as well as access to treatment. They also show lower rates of acceptance of health-promoting behaviours compared with other sectors of society. Thus, policies need to favour the poor and appropriately targeted, as poor people are most at risk and have the least power to effect change.

2.2 The double burden of diseases in the developing world

Hunger and malnutrition remain among the most devastating problems facing the majority of the world's poor and needy people, and continue to dominate the health of the world's poorest nations. Nearly 30% of humanity are currently suffering from one or more of the multiple forms of malnutrition (19).

The tragic consequences of malnutrition include death, disability, stunted mental and physical growth, and as a result, retarded national socioeconomic development. Some 60% of the 10.9 million deaths each year among children aged under five years in the developing world are associated with malnutrition (20). Iodine deficiency is the greatest single preventable cause of brain damage and mental retardation worldwide, and is estimated to affect more than 700 million people, most of them located in the less developed countries (21). Over 2000 million people have iron deficiency anaemia (22). Vitamin A deficiency remains the single greatest preventable cause of needless childhood blindness and increased risk of premature childhood mortality from infectious diseases, with 250 million children under five years of age suffering from subclinical deficiency (23). Intrauterine growth retardation, defined as birth weight below the 10th percentile of the birth-weight-for-gestational-age reference curve, affects 23.8% or approximately 30 million newborn babies per year, profoundly influencing growth, survival, and physical and mental capacity in childhood (24). It also has major public health implications in view of the increased risk of developing diet-related chronic diseases later in life (25–31).

Given the rapidity with which traditional diets and lifestyles are changing in many developing countries, it is not surprising that food insecurity and undernutrition persist in the same countries where chronic diseases are emerging as a major epidemic. The epidemic of obesity, with its attendant comorbidities — heart disease, hypertension, stroke, and diabetes — is not a problem limited to industrialized countries (32). Children are in a similar situation; a disturbing increase in the prevalence of overweight among this group has taken place over the past 20 years in developing countries as diverse as India, Mexico, Nigeria and Tunisia (33). The increasing prevalence of obesity in developing countries also indicates that physical inactivity is an increasing problem in those countries as well.

In the past, undernutrition and chronic diseases were seen as two totally separate problems, despite being present simultaneously. This dichotomy has obstructed effective action to curb the advancing epidemic of chronic diseases. For example, the prevailing approach of measuring child undernutrition on the basis of the underweight indicator (weight-for-age) can lead to gross underestimation of the presence of obesity in populations that have a high prevalence of stunting. Use of this indicator could lead aid programmes to feed apparently underweight people, with the undesirable outcome of further aggravating obesity. In Latin America, close to 90 million people are beneficiaries of food programmes (*34*) but that group actually comprises only 10 million truly underweight people (after correcting for height). The two facets of nutrition-related problems need to be brought together and treated in the context of the whole spectrum of malnutrition.

2.3 An integrated approach to diet-related and nutrition-related diseases

The root causes of malnutrition include poverty and inequity. Eliminating these causes requires political and social action of which nutritional programmes can be only one aspect. Sufficient, safe and varied food supplies not only prevent malnutrition but also reduce the risk of chronic diseases. It is well known that nutritional deficiency increases the risk of common infectious diseases, notably those of childhood, and vice versa (*35, 36*). There is, therefore, complementarity in terms of public health approaches and public policy priorities, between policies and programmes designed to prevent chronic diseases and those designed to prevent other diet-related and nutrition-related diseases.

The double burden of disease is most effectively lifted by a range of integrated policies and programmes. Such an integrated approach is the key to action in countries where modest public health budgets will inevitably remain mostly devoted to prevention of deficiency and infection. Indeed, there is no country, however privileged, in which combating deficiency and infection are no longer public health priorities. High-income countries accustomed to programmes designed to prevent chronic diseases can amplify the effectiveness of the programmes by applying them to the prevention of nutritional deficiency and food-related infectious diseases.

Guidelines designed to give equal priority to the prevention of nutritional deficiency and chronic diseases, have already been established for the Latin American region (*37*). Recent recommendations to prevent cancer are reckoned also to reduce the risk of nutritional deficiency and food-related infectious diseases (*38*), and dietary guide-lines for the Brazilian population give equal priority to the prevention and control of nutritional deficiency, food-related infectious diseases, and chronic diseases (*39*).

References

1. *The world health report 2002: reducing risks, promoting healthy life.* Geneva, World Health Organization, 2002.

2. *Diet, physical activity and health.* Geneva, World Health Organization, 2002 (documents A55/16 and A55/16 Corr.1).

3. **Popkin BM.** The shift in stages of the nutritional transition in the developing world differs from past experiences! *Public Health Nutrition*, 2002, **5**:205–214.

4. *The world health report 1998. Life in the 21st century: a vision for all.* Geneva, World Health Organization, 1998.

5. **Aboderin I et al.** *Life course perspectives on coronary heart disease, stroke and diabetes: key issues and implications for policy and research.* Geneva, World Health Organization, 2001 (document WHO/NMH/NPH/01.4).

6. **Murray CJL, Lopez AD, eds.** *The global burden of disease: a comprehensive assessment of mortality and disability from diseases, injuries, and risk factors in 1990 and projected to 2020.* Cambridge, Harvard School of Public Health on behalf of the World Health Organization and the World Bank, 1996 (Global Burden of Disease and Injury Series, Vol. 1).

7. **Choi BCK, Bonita R, McQueen DV.** The need for global risk factor surveillance. *Journal of Epidemiology and Community Health*, 2001, **55**:370.

8. **Matsudo V et al.** Promotion of physical activity in a developing country: the Agita São Paulo experience. *Public Health Nutrition*, 2002, **5**:253–261.

9. *World declaration and plan of action for nutrition.* Rome, Food and Agriculture Organization of the United Nations and Geneva, World Health Organization, 1992.

10. *Nutrition and development: a global assessment.* Rome, Food and Agriculture Organization of the United Nations and Geneva, World Health Organization, 1992.

11. Promoting appropriate diets and healthy lifestyles. In: *Major issues for nutrition strategies.* Rome, Food and Agriculture Organization of the United Nations and Geneva, World Health Organization, 1992:17–20.

12. Resolution WHA51.12. Health promotion. In: *Fifty-first World Health Assembly, Geneva, 11–16 May 1998. Volume 1. Resolutions and decisions, annexes.* Geneva, World–Health Organization, 1998:11–12 (document WHA51/1998/REC/1).

13. Resolution WHA52.7. Active ageing. In: *Fifty-second World Health Assembly, Geneva, 17–25 May 1999. Volume 1. Resolutions and decisions, annexes.* Geneva, World Health Organization, 1999:8–9 (document WHA52/1999/REC/1).

14. Resolution WHA53.17. Prevention and control of noncommunicable diseases. In: *Fifty-third World Health Assembly, Geneva, 15–20 May 2000. Volume 1. Resolutions and decisions, annex.* Geneva, World Health Organization, 2000:22–24 (document WHA53/2000/REC/1).

15. Resolution WHA53.23. Diet, physical activity and health. In: *Fifty-fifth World Health Assembly, Geneva, 13–18 May 2002. Volume 1. Resolutions and decisions, annexes.* Geneva, World Health Organization, 2002:28–30 (document WHA55/2002/REC/1).

16. Puska P et al. Changes in premature deaths in Finland: successful long-term prevention of cardiovascular diseases. *Bulletin of the World Health Organization*, 1998, 76:419–425.

17. Lee M-J, Popkin BM, Kim S. The unique aspects of the nutrition transition in South Korea: the retention of healthful elements in their traditional diet. *Public Health Nutrition*, 2002, 5:197–203.

18. Kim SW, Moon SJ, Popkin BM. The nutrition transition in South Korea. *American Journal of Clinical Nutrition*, 2002, 71:44–53.

19. *A global agenda for combating malnutrition: progress report.* Geneva, World Health Organization, 2000 (document WHO/NHD/00.6).

20. *Childhood nutrition and progress in implementing the International Code of Marketing of Breast-milk Substitutes.* Geneva, World Health Organization, 2002 (document A55/14).

21. WHO/UNICEF/International Council for the Control of Iodine Deficiency Disorders. *Progress towards the elimination of iodine deficiency disorders (IDD).* Geneva, World Health Organization, 1999 (document WHO/NHD/99.4).

22. WHO/UNICEF/United Nations University. *Iron deficiency anaemia assessment, prevention and control: a guide for programme managers.* Geneva, World Health Organization, 2001 (document WHO/NHD/01.3).

23. WHO/UNICEF. *Global prevalence of vitamin A deficiency. MDIS Working Paper No. 2.* Geneva, World Health Organization, 1995 (document WHO/NUT/95.3).

24. de Onis M, Blössner M, Villar J. Levels and patterns of intrauterine growth retardation in developing countries. *European Journal of Clinical Nutrition*, 1998, 52 (Suppl. 1):S5–S15.

25. Barker DJP et al. Weight in infancy and death from ischaemic heart disease. *Lancet*, 1989, 2:577–580.

26. Barker DJP et al. Type 2 (non-insulin-dependent) diabetes mellitus, hypertension and hyperlipidaemia (syndrome X): relation to reduced fetal growth. *Diabetologia*, 1993, 36:62–67.

27. Barker DJP et al. Growth in utero and serum cholesterol concentrations in adult life. *British Medical Journal*, 1993, 307:1524–1527.

28. Barker DJP. Fetal origins of coronary heart disease. *British Medical Journal*, 1995, 311:171–174.

29. Barker DJP et al. Growth in utero and blood pressure levels in the next generation. *Hypertension*, 2000, 18:843–846.

30. Barker DJP et al. Size at birth and resilience to effects of poor living conditions in adult life: longitudinal study. *British Medical Journal*, 2001, 323:1273–1276.

31. *Programming of chronic disease by impaired fetal nutrition: evidence and implications for policy and intervention strategies.* Geneva, World Health Organization, 2002 (documents WHO/NHD/02.3 and WHO/NPH/02.1).

32. *Obesity: preventing and managing the global epidemic. Report of a WHO Consultation.* Geneva, World Health Organization, 2000 (WHO Technical Report Series, No. 894).

33. de Onis M, Blössner M. Prevalence and trends of overweight among preschool children in developing countries. *American Journal of Clinical Nutrition*, 2000, 72:1032–1039.

34. Peña M, Bacallao J. Obesity among the poor: an emerging problem in Latin America and the Caribbean. In: Peña M, Bacallao J, eds. *Obesity and poverty: a new public health challenge*. Washington, DC, Pan American Health Organization, 2000:3–10 (Scientific Publication, No. 576).

35. Scrimshaw NS, Taylor CE, Gordon JE. *Interactions of nutrition and infection*. Geneva, World Health Organization, 1968.

36. Tompkins A, Watson F. *Malnutrition and infection: a review*. Geneva, Administrative Committee on Coordination/Subcommittee on Nutrition, 1989 (ACC/SCN State-of-the-art Series Nutrition Policy Discussion Paper, No. 5).

37. Bengoa JM et al. *Guiás de alimentacion. [Dietary guidelines.]* Caracas, Fundacion Cavendes, 1988.

38. World Cancer Research Fund/American Institute for Cancer Research. *Food, nutrition and the prevention of cancer: a global perspective*. Washington, DC, American Institute for Cancer Research, 1997:530–534.

39. Ministério da Saúde. *Dietary guidelines for the Brazilian population*. Brasília, Brazilian Ministry of Health (available on the Internet at http://portal.saude.gov.br/alimentacao/english/index.cfm).

3. Global and regional food consumption patterns and trends

3.1 Introduction

Promoting healthy diets and lifestyles to reduce the global burden of noncommunicable diseases requires a multisectoral approach involving the various relevant sectors in societies. The agriculture and food sector figures prominently in this enterprise and must be given due importance in any consideration of the promotion of healthy diets for individuals and population groups. Food strategies must not merely be directed at ensuring food security for all, but must also achieve the consumption of adequate quantities of safe and good quality foods that together make up a healthy diet. Any recommendation to that effect will have implications for all components in the food chain. It is therefore useful at this juncture to examine trends in consumption patterns worldwide and deliberate on the potential of the food and agriculture sector to meet the demands and challenges posed by this report.

Economic development is normally accompanied by improvements in a country's food supply and the gradual elimination of dietary deficiencies, thus improving the overall nutritional status of the country's population. Furthermore, it also brings about qualitative changes in the production, processing, distribution and marketing of food. Increasing urbanization will also have consequences for the dietary patterns and lifestyles of individuals, not all of which are positive. Changes in diets, patterns of work and leisure — often referred to as the "nutrition transition" — are already contributing to the causal factors underlying noncommunicable diseases even in the poorest countries. Moreover, the pace of these changes seems to be accelerating, especially in the low-income and middle-income countries.

The dietary changes that characterize the "nutrition transition" include both quantitative and qualitative changes in the diet. The adverse dietary changes include shifts in the structure of the diet towards a higher energy density diet with a greater role for fat and added sugars in foods, greater saturated fat intake (mostly from animal sources), reduced intakes of complex carbohydrates and dietary fibre, and reduced fruit and vegetable intakes (1). These dietary changes are compounded by lifestyle changes that reflect reduced physical activity at work and during leisure time (2). At the same time, however, poor countries continue to face food shortages and nutrient inadequacies.

Diets evolve over time, being influenced by many factors and complex interactions. Income, prices, individual preferences and beliefs, cultural traditions, as well as geographical, environmental, social and economic factors all interact in a complex manner to shape dietary consumption patterns. Data on the national availability of the main food commodities provide a valuable insight into diets and their evolution over time. FAO produces annual Food Balance Sheets which provide national data on food availability (for almost all commodities and for nearly all countries). Food Balance Sheets give a complete picture of supply (including production, imports, stock changes and exports) and utilization (including final demand in the form of food use and industrial non-food use, intermediate demand such as animal feed and seed use, and waste) by commodity. From these data, the average per capita supply of macronutrients (i.e. energy, protein, fats) can be derived for all food commodities. Although such average per capita supplies are derived from national data, they may not correspond to actual per capita availability, which is determined by many other factors such as inequality in access to food. Likewise, these data refer to "average food available for consumption", which, for a number of reasons (for example, waste at the household level), is not equal to average food intake or average food consumption. In the remainder of this chapter, therefore, the terms "food consumption" or "food intake" should be read as "food available for consumption".

Actual food availability may vary by region, socioeconomic level and season. Certain difficulties are encountered when estimating trade, production and stock changes on an annual scale. Hence three-year averages are calculated in order to reduce errors. The FAO statistical database (FAOSTAT), being based on national data, does not provide information on the distribution of food within countries, or within communities and households.

3.2 Developments in the availability of dietary energy

Food consumption expressed in kilocalories (kcal) per capita per day is a key variable used for measuring and evaluating the evolution of the global and regional food situation. A more appropriate term for this variable would be "national average apparent food consumption" since the data come from national Food Balance Sheets rather than from food consumption surveys. Analysis of FAOSTAT data shows that dietary energy measured in kcals per capita per day has been steadily increasing on a worldwide basis; availability of calories per capita from the mid-1960s to the late 1990s increased globally by approximately 450 kcal per capita per day and by over 600 kcal per capita per day in developing countries (see Table 1). This change has not, however, been equal across regions. The per capita supply of calories has remained almost stagnant in sub-Saharan Africa and has recently fallen in the countries in economic transition. In contrast, the per capita supply of energy has risen dramatically in East Asia (by almost 1000 kcal per capita per day, mainly in China) and in the Near East/North Africa region (by over 700 kcal per capita per day).

Table 1
Global and regional per capita food consumption (kcal per capita per day)

Region	1964–1966	1974–1976	1984–1986	1997–1999	2015	2030
World	2358	2435	2655	2803	2940	3050
Developing countries	2054	2152	2450	2681	2850	2980
Near East and North Africa	2290	2591	2953	3006	3090	3170
Sub-Saharan Africa[a]	2058	2079	2057	2195	2360	2540
Latin America and the Caribbean	2393	2546	2689	2824	2980	3140
East Asia	1957	2105	2559	2921	3060	3190
South Asia	2017	1986	2205	2403	2700	2900
Industrialized countries	2947	3065	3206	3380	3440	3500
Transition countries	3222	3385	3379	2906	3060	3180

[a] Excludes South Africa.

Source: reproduced, with minor editorial amendments from reference 3 with the permission of the publisher.

In short, it would appear that the world has made significant progress in raising food consumption per person. The increase in the world average consumption would have been higher but for the declines in the transition economies that occurred in the 1990s. It is generally agreed, however, that those declines are likely to revert in the near future. The growth in food consumption has been accompanied by significant structural changes and a shift in diet away from staples such as roots and tubers towards more livestock products and vegetable oils (4). Table 1 shows that current energy intakes range from 2681 kcal per capita per day in developing countries, to 2906 kcal per capita per day in transition countries and 3380 kcal per capita per day in industrialized countries. Data shown in Table 2 suggest that per capita energy supply has declined from both animal and vegetable sources in the countries in economic transition, while it has increased in the developing and industrialized countries.

Table 2
Vegetable and animal sources of energy in the diet (kcal per capita per day)

Region	1967–1969			1977–1979			1987–1989			1997–1999		
	T	V	A	T	V	A	T	V	A	T	V	A
Developing countries	2059	1898	161	2254	2070	184	2490	2248	242	2681	2344	337
Transition countries	3287	2507	780	3400	2507	893	3396	2455	941	2906	2235	671
Industrialized countries	3003	2132	871	3112	2206	906	3283	2333	950	3380	2437	943

T, total kcal; V, kcal of vegetable origin; A, kcal of animal origin (including fish products).

Source: FAOSTAT, 2003.

Similar trends are evident for protein availability; this has increased in both developing and industrialized countries but decreased in the transition countries. Although the global supply of protein has been increasing, the distribution of the increase in the protein supply is unequal. The per capita supply of vegetable protein is slightly higher in developing countries, while the supply of animal protein is three times higher in industrialized countries.

Globally, the share of dietary energy supplied by cereals appears to have remained relatively stable over time, representing about 50% of dietary energy supply. Recently, however, subtle changes appear to be taking place (see Fig. 1). A closer analysis of the dietary energy intake shows a decrease in developing countries, where the share of energy derived from cereals has fallen from 60% to 54% in a period of only 10 years. Much of this downwards trend is attributable to cereals, particularly wheat and rice, becoming less preferred foods in middle-income countries such as Brazil and China, a pattern likely to continue over the next 30 years or so. Fig. 2 shows the structural changes in the diet of developing countries over the past 30–40 years and FAO's projections to the year 2030 (3).

Figure 1
The share of dietary energy derived from cereals

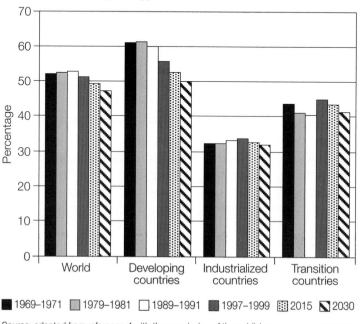

1969–1971　1979–1981　1989–1991　1997–1999　2015　2030

Source: adapted from reference 4 with the permission of the publisher.　WHO 03.19

Figure 2
Calories from major commodities in developing countries

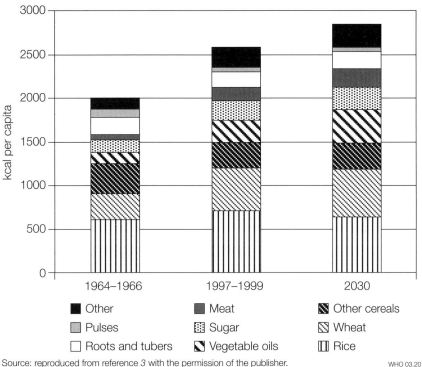

Source: reproduced from reference *3* with the permission of the publisher.   WHO 03.20

3.3 Availability and changes in consumption of dietary fat

The increase in the quantity and quality of the fats consumed in the diet is an important feature of nutrition transition reflected in the national diets of countries. There are large variations across the regions of the world in the amount of total fats (i.e. fats in foods, plus added fats and oils) available for human consumption. The lowest quantities consumed are recorded in Africa, while the highest consumption occurs in parts of North America and Europe. The important point is that there has been a remarkable increase in the intake of dietary fats over the past three decades (see Table 3) and that this increase has taken place practically everywhere except in Africa, where consumption levels have stagnated. The per capita supply of fat from animal foods has increased, respectively, by 14 and 4 g per capita in developing and industrialized countries, while there has been a decrease of 9 g per capita in transition countries.

Table 3
Trends in the dietary supply of fat

Region	Supply of fat (g per capita per day)				
	1967–1969	1977–1979	1987–1989	1997–1999	Change between 1967-1969 and 1997-1999
World	53	57	67	73	20
North Africa	44	58	65	64	20
Sub-Saharan Africa[a]	41	43	41	45	4
North America	117	125	138	143	26
Latin America and the Caribbean	54	65	73	79	25
China	24	27	48	79	55
East and South-East Asia	28	32	44	52	24
South Asia	29	32	39	45	16
European Community	117	128	143	148	31
Eastern Europe	90	111	116	104	14
Near East	51	62	73	70	19
Oceania	102	102	113	113	11

[a] Excludes South Africa
Source: FAOSTAT, 2003.

The increase in dietary fat supply worldwide exceeds the increase in dietary protein supply. The average global supply of fat has increased by 20 g per capita per day since 1967–1969. This increase in availability has been most pronounced in the Americas, East Asia, and the European Community. The proportion of energy contributed by dietary fats exceeds 30% in the industrialized regions, and in nearly all other regions this share is increasing.

The fat-to-energy ratio (FER) is defined as the percentage of energy derived from fat in the total supply of energy (in kcal). Country-specific analysis of FAO data for 1988–1990 (5) found a range for the FER of 7–46%. A total of 19 countries fell below the minimum recommendation of 15% dietary energy supply from fat, the majority of these being in sub-Saharan Africa and the remainder in South Asia. In contrast, 24 countries were above the maximum recommendation of 35%, the majority of these countries being in North America and Western Europe. It is useful to note that limitations of the Food Balance Sheet data may contribute much of this variation in the FER between countries. For instance, in countries such as Malaysia with abundant availability of vegetable oils at low prices, Food Balance Sheet data may not reflect real consumption at the individual household level.

Rising incomes in the developing world have also led to an increase in the availability and consumption of energy-dense high-fat diets. Food balance data can be used to examine the shift in the proportion of energy from fat over time and its relationship to increasing incomes (6).

In 1961–1963, a diet providing 20% of energy from fat was associated only with countries having at least a per capita gross national product of US$ 1475. By 1990, however, even poor countries having a gross national product of only US$ 750 per capita had access to a similar diet comprising 20% of energy from fat. (Both values of gross national product are given in 1993 US$.) This change was mainly the result of an increase in the consumption of vegetable fats by poor countries, with smaller increases occurred in middle-income and high-income countries. By 1990, vegetable fats accounted for a greater proportion of dietary energy than animal fats for countries in the lowest per capita income category. Changes in edible vegetable oil supply, in prices and in consumption equally affected rich and poor countries, although the net impact was relatively much greater in low-income countries. An equally large and important shift in the proportion of energy from added sugars in the diets of low-income countries was also a feature of the nutrition transition (1).

Examinations of the purchasing habits of people, aimed at understanding the relationship between level of education or income and the different amounts or types of commodities purchased at different times were also revealing. Research conducted in China shows that there have been profound shifts in purchasing practices in relation to income over the past decade. These analyses show how extra income in China affects poor people and rich people in a differential manner, enhancing the fat intake of the poor more than that of the rich (7).

A variable proportion of these fat calories are provided by saturated fatty acids. Only in the two of the most affluent regions (i.e. in parts of North America and Europe) is the intake of saturated fat at or above 10% of energy intake level. In other less affluent regions, the proportion of dietary energy contributed by saturated fatty acids is lower, ranging from 5% to 8%, and generally not changing much over time. National dietary surveys conducted in some countries confirm these data. The ratio of dietary fat from animal sources to total fat is a key indicator, since foods from animal sources are high in saturated fat. Data sets used to calculate country-specific FERs can also be used to calculate proportions of animal fat in total fat. Such analysis indicated that the proportion of animal fat in total fat was lower than 10% in some countries (Democratic Republic of Congo, Mozambique, Nigeria, Sao Tome and Principe, and Sierra Leone), while it is above 75% in some other countries (Denmark, Finland, Hungary, Mongolia, Poland and Uruguay). These findings are not strictly divided along economic lines, as not all of the countries in the high range represent the most affluent countries. Country-specific food availability and cultural dietary preferences and norms to some extent determine these patterns.

The types of edible oils used in developing countries are also changing with the increasing use of hardened margarines (rich in trans fatty acids) that do not need to be refrigerated. Palm oil is becoming an increasingly important edible oil in the diets of much of South-East Asia and is likely to be a major source in the coming years. Currently, palm oil consumption is low and the FER ranges between 15% and 18%. At this low level of consumption, the saturated fatty acid content of the diet comprises only 4% to 8%. Potential developments in the edible oil sector could affect all stages of the oil production process from plant breeding to processing methods, including the blending of oils aimed at producing edible oils that have a healthy fatty acid composition.

Olive oil is an important edible oil consumed largely in the Mediterranean region. Its production has been driven by rising demand, which has increasingly shifted olive cultivation from traditional farms to more intensive forms of cultivation. There is some concern that the intensive cultivation of olives may have adverse environmental impacts, such as soil erosion and desertification (8). However, agricultural production methods are being developed to ensure less harmful impacts on the environment.

3.4 Availability and changes in consumption of animal products

There has been an increasing pressure on the livestock sector to meet the growing demand for high-value animal protein. The world's livestock sector is growing at an unprecedented rate and the driving force behind this enormous surge is a combination of population growth, rising incomes and urbanization. Annual meat production is projected to increase from 218 million tonnes in 1997–1999 to 376 million tonnes by 2030.

There is a strong positive relationship between the level of income and the consumption of animal protein, with the consumption of meat, milk and eggs increasing at the expense of staple foods. Because of the recent steep decline in prices, developing countries are embarking on higher meat consumption at much lower levels of gross domestic product than the industrialized countries did some 20–30 years ago.

Urbanization is a major driving force influencing global demand for livestock products. Urbanization stimulates improvements in infrastructure, including cold chains, which permit trade in perishable goods. Compared with the less diversified diets of the rural communities, city dwellers have a varied diet rich in animal proteins and fats, and characterized by higher consumption of meat, poultry, milk and other dairy products. Table 4 shows trends in per capita consumption of livestock products in different regions and country groups. There has been a remarkable increase in the consumption of animal products in countries such as Brazil and China, although the levels are still well below the levels of consumption in North American and most other industrialized countries.

As diets become richer and more diverse, the high-value protein that the livestock sector offers improves the nutrition of the vast majority of the world. Livestock products not only provide high-value protein but are also important sources of a wide range of essential micronutrients, in particular minerals such as iron and zinc, and vitamins such as vitamin A. For the large majority of people in the world, particularly in developing countries, livestock products remain a desired food for nutritional value and taste. Excessive consumption of animal products in some countries and social classes can, however, lead to excessive intakes of fat.

Table 4
Per capita consumption of livestock products

Region	Meat (kg per year)			Milk (kg per year)		
	1964–1966	1997–1999	2030	1964–1966	1997–1999	2030
World	24.2	36.4	45.3	73.9	78.1	89.5
Developing countries	10.2	25.5	36.7	28.0	44.6	65.8
Near East and North Africa	11.9	21.2	35.0	68.6	72.3	89.9
Sub-Saharan Africa[a]	9.9	9.4	13.4	28.5	29.1	33.8
Latin America and the Caribbean	31.7	53.8	76.6	80.1	110.2	139.8
East Asia	8.7	37.7	58.5	3.6	10.0	17.8
South Asia	3.9	5.3	11.7	37.0	67.5	106.9
Industrialized countries	61.5	88.2	100.1	185.5	212.2	221.0
Transition countries	42.5	46.2	60.7	156.6	159.1	178.7

[a] Excludes South Africa.

Source: Adapted from reference 4 with the permission of the publisher.

The growing demand for livestock products is likely to have an undesirable impact on the environment. For example, there will be more large-scale, industrial production, often located close to urban centres, which brings with it a range of environmental and public health risks. Attempts have been made to estimate the environmental impact of industrial livestock production. For instance, it has been estimated that the number of people fed in a year per hectare ranges from 22 for potatoes and 19 for rice to 1 and 2, respectively, for beef and lamb (9). The low energy conversion ratio from feed to meat is another concern, since some of the cereal grain food produced is diverted to livestock production. Likewise, land and water requirements for meat production are likely to become a major concern, as the increasing demand for animal products results in more intensive livestock production systems (10).

3.5 Availability and consumption of fish

Despite fluctuations in supply and demand caused by the changing state of fisheries resources, the economic climate and environmental conditions, fisheries, including aquaculture, have traditionally been, and remain an important source of food, employment and revenue in many countries and communities (*11*). After the remarkable increase in both marine and inland capture of fish during the 1950s and 1960s, world fisheries production has levelled off since the 1970s. This levelling off of the total catch follows the general trend of most of the world's fishing areas, which have apparently reached their maximum potential for fisheries production, with the majority of stocks being fully exploited. It is therefore very unlikely that substantial increases in total catch will be obtained in the future. In contrast, aquaculture production has followed the opposite path. Starting from an insignificant total production, inland and marine aquaculture production has been growing at a remarkable rate, offsetting part of the reduction in the ocean catch of fish.

The total food fish supply and hence consumption has been growing at a rate of 3.6% per year since 1961, while the world's population has been expanding at 1.8% per year. The proteins derived from fish, crustaceans and molluscs account for between 13.8% and 16.5% of the animal protein intake of the human population. The average apparent per capita consumption increased from about 9 kg per year in the early 1960s to 16 kg in 1997. The per capita availability of fish and fishery products has therefore nearly doubled in 40 years, outpacing population growth.

As well as income-related variations, the role of fish in nutrition shows marked continental, regional and national differences. In industrialized countries, where diets generally contain a more diversified range of animal proteins, a rise in per capita provision from 19.7 kg to 27.7 kg seems to have occurred. This represents a growth rate close to 1% per year. In this group of countries, fish contributed an increasing share of total protein intake until 1989 (accounting for between 6.5% and 8.5%), but since then its importance has gradually declined and, in 1997, its percentage contribution was back to the level prevailing in the mid-1980s. In the early 1960s, per capita fish supply in low-income food-deficit countries was, on average, only 30% of that of the richest countries. This gap has been gradually reduced, such that in 1997, average fish consumption in these countries was 70% of that of the more affluent economies. Despite the relatively low consumption by weight in low-income food-deficit countries, the contribution of fish to total animal protein intake is considerable (nearly 20%). Over the past four decades, however, the share of fish proteins in animal proteins has declined slightly, because of faster growth in the consumption of other animal products.

Currently, two-thirds of the total food fish supply is obtained from capture fisheries in marine and inland waters, while the remaining one-third is derived from aquaculture. The contribution of inland and marine capture fisheries to per capita food supply has stabilized, around 10 kg per capita in the period 1984–1998. Any recent increases in per capita availability have, therefore, been obtained from aquaculture production, from both traditional rural aquaculture and intensive commercial aquaculture of high-value species.

Fish contributes up to 180 kcal per capita per day, but reaches such high levels only in a few countries where there is a lack of alternative protein foods grown locally or where there is a strong preference for fish (examples are Iceland, Japan and some small island states). More typically, fish provides about 20–30 kcal per capita per day. Fish proteins are essential in the diet of some densely populated countries where the total protein intake level is low, and are very important in the diets of many other countries. Worldwide, about a billion people rely on fish as their main source of animal proteins. Dependence on fish is usually higher in coastal than in inland areas. About 20% of the world's population derives at least one-fifth of its animal protein intake from fish, and some small island states depend almost exclusively on fish.

Recommending the increased consumption of fish is another area where the feasibility of dietary recommendations needs to be balanced against concerns for sustainability of marine stocks and the potential depletion of this important marine source of high quality nutritious food. Added to this is the concern that a significant proportion of the world fish catch is transformed into fish meal and used as animal feed in industrial livestock production and thus is not available for human consumption.

3.6 Availability and consumption of fruits and vegetables

Consumption of fruits and vegetables plays a vital role in providing a diversified and nutritious diet. A low consumption of fruits and vegetables in many regions of the developing world is, however, a persistent phenomenon, confirmed by the findings of food consumption surveys. Nationally representative surveys in India (12), for example, indicate a steady level of consumption of only 120–140 g per capita per day, with about another 100 g per capita coming from roots and tubers, and some 40 g per capita from pulses. This may not be true for urban populations in India, who have rising incomes and greater access to a diverse and varied diet. In contrast, in China, – a country that is undergoing rapid economic growth and transition – the amount of fruits and vegetables consumed has increased to 369 g per capita per day by 1992.

At present, only a small and negligible minority of the world's population consumes the generally recommended high average intake of fruits and vegetables. In 1998, only 6 of the 14 WHO regions had an availability of fruits and vegetables equal to or greater than the earlier recommended intake of 400 g per capita per day. The relatively favourable situation in 1998 appears to have evolved from a markedly less favourable position in previous years, as evidenced by the great increase in vegetable availability recorded between 1990 and 1998 for most of the regions. In contrast, the availability of fruit generally decreased between 1990 and 1998 in most regions of the world.

The increase in urbanization globally is another challenge. Increasing urbanization will distance more people from primary food production, and in turn have a negative impact on both the availability of a varied and nutritious diet with enough fruits and vegetables, and the access of the urban poor to such a diet. Nevertheless, it may facilitate the achievement of other goals, as those who can afford it can have better access to a diverse and varied diet. Investment in periurban horticulture may provide an opportunity to increase the availability and consumption of a healthy diet.

Global trends in the production and supply of vegetables indicate that the current production and consumption vary widely among regions, as indicated in Table 5. It should be noted that the production of wild and indigenous vegetables is not taken into account in production statistics and might therefore be underestimated in consumption statistics. In 2000, the global annual average per capita vegetable supply was 102 kg, with the highest level in Asia (116 kg), and the lowest levels in South America (48 kg) and Africa (52 kg). These figures also include the large amount of horticultural produce that is consumed on the farm. Table 5 and Figure 3 illustrate the regional and temporal variations in the per capita availability of vegetables per capita over the past few decades.

Table 5
Supply of vegetables per capita, by region, 1979 and 2000 (kg per capita per year)

Region	1979	2000
World	66.1	101.9
Developed countries	107.4	112.8
Developing countries	51.1	98.8
Africa	45.4	52.1
North and Central America	88.7	98.3
South America	43.2	47.8
Asia	56.6	116.2
Europe	110.9	112.5
Oceania	71.8	98.7

Source: reproduced from reference *13* with the permission of the publisher.

Figure 3

Trends in the supply of vegetables per capita, by region, 1970–2000

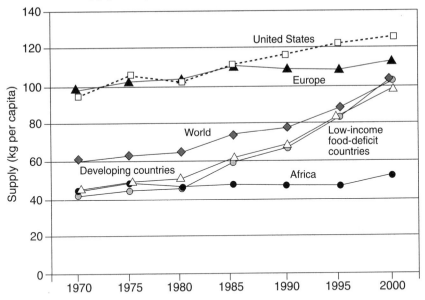

Source: reproduced from reference *13* with the permission of the publisher.

WHO 03.21

3.7 Future trends in demand, food availability and consumption

In recent years the growth rates of world agricultural production and crop yields have slowed. This has raised fears that the world may not be able to grow enough food and other commodities to ensure that future populations are adequately fed. However, the slowdown has occurred not because of shortages of land or water but rather because demand for agricultural products has also slowed. This is mainly because world population growth rates have been declining since the late 1960s, and fairly high levels of food consumption per person are now being reached in many countries, beyond which further rises will be limited. It also true that a high share of the world's population remains in poverty and hence lacks the necessary income to translate its needs into effective demand. As a result, the growth in world demand for agricultural products is expected to fall from an average 2.2% per year over the past 30 years to an average 1.5% per year for the next 30 years. In developing countries the slowdown will be more dramatic, from 3.7% per year to 2% per year, partly as a result of China having passed the phase of rapid growth in its demand for food. Global food shortages are unlikely, but serious problems already exist at national and local levels, and may worsen unless focused efforts are made.

The annual growth rate of world demand for cereals has declined from 2.5% per year in the 1970s and 1.9% per year in the 1980s to only 1% per year in the 1990s. Annual cereal use per person (including animal feeds) peaked in the mid-1980s at 334 kg and has since fallen to 317 kg. The decline is not a cause for alarm, it is largely the natural result of slower population growth and shifts in human diets and animal feeds. During the 1990s, however, the decline was accentuated by a number of temporary factors, including serious economic recessions in the transition countries and in some East and South-East Asian countries.

The growth rate in the demand for cereals is expected to rise again to 1.4% per year up until 2015, slowing to 1.2% per year thereafter. In developing countries overall, cereal production is not expected to keep pace with demand. The net cereal deficits of these countries, which amounted to 103 million tonnes or 9% of consumption in 1997–1999, could rise to 265 million tonnes by 2030, when they will be 14% of consumption. This gap can be bridged by increased surpluses from traditional grain exporters, and by new exports from the transition countries, which are expected to shift from being net importers to being net exporters.

Oil crops have seen the fastest increase in area of any crop sector, expanding by 75 million hectares between the mid-1970s and the end of the 1990s, while cereal area fell by 28 million hectares over the same period. Future per capita consumption of oil crops is expected to rise more rapidly than that of cereals. These crops will account for 45 out of every 100 extra kilocalories added to average diets in developing countries between now and 2030.

There are three main sources of growth in crop production: expanding the land area, increasing the frequency at which it is cropped (often through irrigation), and boosting yields. It has been suggested that growth in crop production may be approaching the ceiling of what is possible in respect of all three sources. A detailed examination of production potentials does not support this view at the global level, although in some countries, and even in whole regions, serious problems already exist and could deepen.

Diets in developing countries are changing as incomes rise. The share of staples, such as cereals, roots and tubers, is declining, while that of meat, dairy products and oil crops is rising. Between 1964–1966 and 1997–1999, per capita meat consumption in developing countries rose by 150% and that of milk and dairy products by 60%. By 2030, per capita consumption of livestock products could rise by a further 44%. Poultry consumption is predicted to grow the fastest. Productivity improvements are likely to be a major source of growth. Milk yields should improve, while breeding and improved management should increase average carcass weights and off-take rates. This will allow increased production with lower growth in animal numbers, and a corresponding slowdown in the growth of environmental damage from grazing and animal wastes.

In developing countries, demand is predicted to grow faster than production, resulting in a growing trade deficit. In meat products this deficit will rise steeply, from 1.2 million tonnes per year in 1997–1999 to 5.9 million tonnes per year in 2030 (despite growing meat exports from Latin America), while in the case of milk and dairy products, the rise will be less steep but still considerable, from 20 million tonnes per year in 1997–1999 to 39 million tonnes per year in 2030. An increasing share of livestock production will probably come from industrial enterprises. In recent years, production from this sector has grown twice as fast as that from more traditional mixed farming systems and more than six times faster than that from grazing systems.

World fisheries production has kept ahead of population growth over the past three decades. Total fish production has almost doubled, from 65 million tonnes in 1970 to 125 million tonnes in 1999, when the world average intake of fish, crustaceans and molluscs reached 16.3 kg per person. By 2030, annual fish consumption is likely to rise to some 150–160 million tonnes, or between 19–20 kg per person. This amount is significantly lower than the potential demand, as environmental factors are expected to limit supply. During the 1990s the marine catch levelled out at 80–85 million tonnes per year, and by the turn of the century, three-quarters of ocean fish stocks were overfished, depleted or exploited up to their maximum sustainable yield. Further growth in the marine catch can only be modest.

Aquaculture compensated for this marine slowdown, doubling its share of world fish production during the 1990s. It is expected to continue to grow rapidly, at rates of 5–7% per year up to 2015. In all sectors of fishing it will be essential to pursue forms of management conducive to sustainable exploitation, especially for resources under common ownership or no ownership.

3.8 Conclusions

A number of conclusions can be drawn from the preceding discussion.

- Most of the information on food consumption has hitherto been obtained from national Food Balance Sheet data. In order to better understand the relationship between food consumption patterns, diets and the emergence of noncommunicable diseases, it is crucial to obtain more reliable information on actual food consumption patterns and trends based on representative consumption surveys.

- There is a need to monitor how the recommendations in this report influence the behaviour of consumers, and what further action is needed to change their diets (and lifestyles) towards more healthy patterns.
- The implications for agriculture, livestock, fisheries and horticulture will have to be assessed and action taken to deal with potential future demands of an increasing and more affluent population. To meet the specified levels of consumption, new strategies may need to be developed. For example, a realistic approach to the implementation of the recommendation concerning high average intake of fruit and vegetables, requires attention to be paid to crucial matters such as where would the large quantities needed be produced, how can the infrastructure be developed to permit trade in these perishable products, and would large-scale production of horticultural products be sustainable?
- A number of more novel matters will need to be dealt with, such as:
  - the positive and negative impacts on noncommunicable diseases of intensive production systems, not only in terms of health (e.g. nitrite in vegetables, heavy metals in irrigation water and manure, pesticide use), but also in terms of dietary quality (e.g. leaner meats in intensive poultry production);
  - the effects of longer food chains, in particular of longer storage and transport routes, such as the higher risk of deterioration (even if most of this may be bacterial and hence not a factor in chronic diseases), and the use and misuse of conserving agents and contaminants;
  - the effects of changes in varietal composition and diversity of consumption patterns, for example, the loss of traditional crop varieties and, perhaps even more significantly, the declining use of foods from "wild" sources.
- Trade aspects need to be considered in the context of improving diet, nutrition and the prevention of chronic diseases. Trade has an important role to play in improving food and nutrition security. On the import side, lower trade barriers reduce domestic food prices, increase the purchasing power of consumers and afford them a greater variety of food products. Freer trade can thus help enhance the availability and affordability of food and contribute to a better-balanced diet. On the export side, access to markets abroad creates new income opportunities for domestic farmers and food processors. Farmers in developing countries in particular stand to benefit from the removal of trade barriers for commodities such as sugar, fruits and vegetables, as well as tropical beverages, all these being products for which they have a comparative advantage.
- The impact that agricultural policies, particularly subsidies, have on the structure of production, processing and marketing systems — and

ultimately on the availability of foods that support healthy food consumption patterns — should not be overlooked.

All these issues and challenges need to be addressed in a pragmatic and intersectoral manner. All sectors in the food chain, from "farm to table", will need to be involved if the food system is to respond to the challenges posed by the need for changes in diets to cope with the burgeoning epidemic of noncommunicable diseases.

References

1. Drewnowski A, Popkin BM. The nutrition transition: new trends in the global diet. *Nutrition Reviews*, 1997, **55**:31–43.

2. Ferro-Luzzi A, Martino L. Obesity and physical activity. *Ciba Foundation Symposium*, 1996, **201**:207–221.

3. *World agriculture: towards 2015/2030. Summary report.* Rome, Food and Agriculture Organization of the United Nations, 2002.

4. Bruinsma J, ed. *World agriculture: towards 2015/2030. An FAO perspective.* Rome, Food and Agriculture Organization of the United Nations/London, Earthscan, 2003.

5. *Fats and oils in human nutrition. Report of a Joint Expert Consultation.* Rome, Food and Agriculture Organization of the United Nations, 1994 (FAO Food and Nutrition Paper, No. 57).

6. Guo X et al. Structural change in the impact of income on food consumption in China 1989–1993. *Economic Development and Cultural Change*, 2000, **48**:737–760.

7. Popkin BM. Nutrition in transition: the changing global nutrition challenge. *Asia Pacific Journal of Clinical Nutrition*, 2001, **10**(Suppl. 1):S13–S18.

8. Beaufoy G. *The environmental impact of olive oil production in the European Union: practical options for improving the environmental impact.* Brussels, Environment Directorate-General, European Commission, 2000.

9. Spedding CRW. The effect of dietary changes on agriculture. In: Lewis B, Assmann G, eds. *The social and economic contexts of coronary prevention.* London, Current Medical Literature, 1990.

10. Pimental D et al. Water resources: agriculture, the environment and society. *Bioscience,* 1997, **47**:97–106.

11. *The state of the world fisheries and aquaculture 2002.* Rome, Food and Agriculture Organization of the United Nations, 2002.

12. *India nutrition profile 1998.* New Delhi, Department of Women and Child Development, Ministry of Human Resource Development, Government of India, 1998.

13. Fresco LO, Baudoin WO. Food and nutrition security towards human security. In: *Proceedings of the International Conference on Vegetables, (ICV-2002), 11–14 November 2002, Bangalore, India.* Bangalore, Dr Prem Nath Agricultural Science Foundation (in press).

4. Diet, nutrition and chronic diseases in context

4.1 Introduction

The diets people eat, in all their cultural variety, define to a large extent people's health, growth and development. Risk behaviours, such as tobacco use and physical inactivity, modify the result for better or worse. All this takes place in a social, cultural, political and economic environment that can aggravate the health of populations unless active measures are taken to make the environment a health-promoting one.

Although this report has taken a disease approach for convenience, the Expert Consultation was mindful in all its discussions that diet, nutrition and physical activity do not take place in a vacuum. Since the publication of the earlier report in 1990 (1), there have been great advances in basic research, considerable expansion of knowledge, and much community and international experience in the prevention and control of chronic diseases. At the same time, the human genome has been mapped and must now enter any discussion of chronic disease.

Concurrently there has been a return to the concept of the basic life course, i.e. of the continuity of human lives from fetus to old age. The influences in the womb work differently from later influences, but clearly have a strong effect on the subsequent manifestation of chronic disease. The known risk factors are now recognized as being amenable to alleviation throughout life, even into old age. The continuity of the life course is seen in the way that both undernutrition and overnutrition (as well as a host of other factors) play a role in the development of chronic disease. The effects of man-made and natural environments (and the interaction between the two) on the development of chronic diseases are increasingly recognized. Such factors are also being recognized as happening further and further "upstream" in the chain of events predisposing humans to chronic disease. All these broadening perceptions not only give a clearer picture of what is happening in the current epidemic of chronic diseases, but also present many opportunities to address them. The identities of those affected are now better recognized: those most disadvantaged in more affluent countries, and – in numerical terms far greater – the populations of the developing and transitional worlds.

There is a continuity in the influences contributing to chronic disease development, and thus also to the opportunities for prevention. These influences include the life course; the microscopic environment of the gene to macroscopic urban and rural environments; the impact of social and political events in one sphere affecting the health and diet of populations far distant; and the way in which already stretched agriculture and oceanic systems will affect the choices available and the recommendations that can be made. For chronic diseases, risks occur at all ages; conversely, all ages are part of the continuum of opportunities for their prevention and control. Both undernutrition and overnutrition are negative influences in terms of disease development, and possibly a combination is even worse; consequently the developing world needs additional targeting. Those with least power need different preventive approaches from the more affluent. Work has to start with the individual risk factors, but, critically, attempts at prevention and health promotion must also take account of the wider social, political and economic environment. Economics, industry, consumer groups and advertising all must be included in the prevention equation.

4.2 Diet, nutrition and the prevention of chronic diseases through the life course

The rapidly increasing burden of chronic diseases is a key determinant of global public health. Already 79% of deaths attributable to chronic diseases are occurring in developing countries, predominantly in middle-aged men (2). There is increasing evidence that chronic disease risks begin in fetal life and continue into old age (3–9). Adult chronic disease, therefore, reflects cumulative differential lifetime exposures to damaging physical and social environments.

For these reasons a life-course approach that captures both the cumulative risk and the many opportunities to intervene that this affords, was adopted by the Expert Consultation. While accepting the imperceptible progression from one life stage to the next, five stages were identified for convenience. These are: fetal development and the maternal environment; infancy; childhood and adolescence; adulthood; and ageing and older people.

4.2.1 Fetal development and the maternal environment

The four relevant factors in fetal life are: (i) intrauterine growth retardation (IUGR); (ii) premature delivery of a normal growth for gestational age fetus; (iii) overnutrition in utero; and (iv) intergenerational factors. There is considerable evidence, mostly from developed countries, that IUGR is associated with an increased risk of coronary heart disease, stroke, diabetes and raised blood pressure (9–20). It may rather be the pattern of growth, i.e. restricted fetal growth followed by very rapid postnatal catch-up growth, that is important in the underlying disease pathways. On the other hand, large size at birth (macrosomia) is also associated with an increased risk of diabetes and cardiovascular disease (16, 21). Among the adult population in India, an association was found between impaired glucose tolerance and high ponderal index (i.e. fatness) at birth (22). In Pima Indians, a U-shaped relationship to birth weight was found, whereas no such relationship was found amongst Mexican Americans (*21, 23*). Higher birth weight has also been related to an increased risk of breast and other cancers (*24*).

In sum, the evidence suggests that optimal birth weight and length distribution should be considered, not only in terms of immediate morbidity and mortality but also in regard to long-term outcomes such as susceptibility to diet-related chronic disease later in life.

4.2.2 *Infancy*

Retarded growth in infancy can be a reflected in a failure to gain weight and a failure to gain height. Both retarded growth and excessive weight or height gain ("crossing the centiles") can be factors in later incidence of chronic disease. An association between low growth in early infancy (low weight at 1 year) and an increased risk of coronary heart disease (CHD) has been described, irrespective of size at birth (*3, 25*). Blood pressure has been found to be highest in those with retarded fetal growth and greater weight gain in infancy (*26*). Short stature, a reflection of socioeconomic deprivation in childhood (*27*), is also associated with an increased risk of CHD and stroke, and to some extent, diabetes (*10, 15, 28–34*). The risk of stroke, and also of cancer mortality at several sites, including breast, uterus and colon, is increased if shorter children display an accelerated growth in height (*35, 36*).

Breastfeeding

There is increasing evidence that among term and pre-term infants, breastfeeding is associated with significantly lower blood pressure levels in childhood (*37, 38*). Consumption of formula instead of breast milk in infancy has also been shown to increase diastolic and mean arterial blood pressure in later life (*37*). Nevertheless, studies with older cohorts (*22*) and the Dutch study of famine (*39*) have not identified such associations. There is increasingly strong evidence suggesting that a lower risk of developing obesity (*40–43*) may be directly related to length of exclusive breastfeeding although it may not become evident until later in childhood (*44*). Some of the discrepancy may be explained by socioeconomic and maternal education factors confounding the findings.

Data from most, but not all, observational studies of term infants have generally suggested adverse effects of formula consumption on the other risk factors for cardiovascular disease (as well as blood pressure), but little information to support this finding is available from controlled clinical trials (*45*). Nevertheless, the weight of current evidence indicates adverse effects of formula milk on cardiovascular disease risk factors; this is consistent with the observations of increased mortality among older adults who were fed formula as infants (*45–47*). The risk for several chronic diseases of childhood and adolescence (e.g. type 1 diabetes, coeliac disease, some childhood cancers, inflammatory bowel disease) have also been associated with infant feeding on breast-milk substitutes and short-term breastfeeding (48).

There has been great interest in the possible effect of high-cholesterol feeding in early life. Reiser et al. (49) proposed the hypothesis that high-cholesterol feeding in early life may serve to regulate cholesterol and lipoprotein metabolism in later life. Animal data in support of this hypothesis are limited, but the idea of a possible metabolic imprinting served to trigger several retrospective and prospective studies in which cholesterol and lipoprotein metabolism in infants fed human milk were compared with those fed formula. Studies in suckling rats have suggested that the presence of cholesterol in the early diet may serve to define a metabolic pattern for lipoproteins and plasma cholesterol that could be of benefit later in life. The study by Mott, Lewis & McGill (50) on differential diets in infant baboons, however, provided evidence to the contrary in terms of benefit. Nevertheless, the observation of modified responses of adult cholesterol production rates, bile cholesterol saturation indices, and bile acid turnover, depending on whether the baboons were fed breast milk or formula, served to attract further interest. It was noted that increased atherosclerotic lesions associated with increased levels of plasma total cholesterol were related to increased dietary cholesterol in early life. No long-term human morbidity and mortality data supporting this notion have been reported.

Short-term human studies have been in part confounded by diversity in solid food weaning regimens, as well as by the varied composition of fatty acid components of the early diet. The latter are now known to have an impact on circulating lipoprotein cholesterol species (51). Mean plasma total cholesterol by age 4 months in infants fed breast milk reached 180 mg/dl or greater, while cholesterol values in infants fed formula tended to remain under 150 mg/dl. In a study by Carlson, DeVoe & Barness (52), infants receiving predominantly a linoleic acid-enriched oil blend exhibited a mean cholesterol concentration of approximately 110 mg/dl. A separate group of infants in that study who received predominantly oleic acid had a mean cholesterol concentration of 133 mg/dl. Moreover, infants who were fed breast milk and oleic acid-enriched formula had higher high-density lipoprotein (HDL) cholesterol and apoproteins A-I and A-II than the predominantly linoleic acid-enriched oil diet group. The ratio of low-density lipoprotein (LDL) cholesterol plus very low-density lipoprotein (VLDL) cholesterol to HDL cholesterol was lowest for infants receiving the formula in which oleic acid was predominant. Using a similar oleic acid predominant formula, Darmady, Fosbrooke & Lloyd (53) reported a mean value of 149 mg/dl at age 4 months, compared with 196 mg/dl in a parallel breast-fed group. Most of those infants then received an uncontrolled mixed diet and cow's milk, with no evident differences in plasma cholesterol levels by 12 months, independent of the type of early feeding they had received. A more recent controlled study (54) suggests that the specific fatty acid intake plays a predominant role in determining total and LDL cholesterol. The significance of high dietary cholesterol associated with exclusive human milk feeding during the first 4 months of life has no demonstrated adverse effect. Measurements of serum lipoprotein concentrations and LDL receptor activity in infants suggests that it is the fatty acid content rather than the cholesterol in the diet which regulates cholesterol homeostasis. The regulation of endogenous cholesterol synthesis in infants appears to be regulated in a similar manner to that of adults (55, 56).

4.2.3 *Childhood and adolescence*

An association between low growth in childhood and an increased risk of CHD has been described, irrespective of size at birth (3, 25). Although based only on developed country research at this point, this finding gives credence to the importance that is currently attached to the role of immediate postnatal factors in shaping disease risk. Growth rates in infants in Bangladesh, most of whom had chronic intrauterine under-nourishment and were breastfed, were similar to growth rates of breastfed infants in industrialized countries, but catch-up growth was limited and weight at 12 months was largely a function of weight at birth (57).

In a study of 11–12 year-old Jamaican children (26), blood pressure levels were found to be highest in those with retarded fetal growth and greater weight gain between the ages of 7 and 11 years. Similar results were found in India (58). Low birth weight Indian babies have been described as having a characteristic poor muscle but high fat preservation, so-called "thin-fat" babies. This phenotype persists throughout the postnatal period and is associated with an increased central adiposity in childhood that is linked to the highest risk of raised blood pressure and disease (59–61). In most studies, the association between low birth weight and high blood pressure has been found to be particularly strong if adjusted to current body size — body mass index (BMI) — suggesting the importance of weight gain after birth (62).

Relative weight in adulthood and weight gain have been found to be associated with increased risk of cancer of the breast, colon, rectum, prostate and other sites (36). Whether there is an independent effect of childhood weight is difficult to determine, as childhood overweight is usually continued into adulthood. Relative weight in adolescence was significantly associated with colon cancer in one retrospective cohort study (63). Frankel, Gunnel & Peters (64), in the follow-up to an earlier survey by Boyd Orr in the late 1930s, found that for both sexes, after accounting for the confounding effects of social class, there was a significant positive relationship between childhood energy intake and adult cancer mortality. The recent review by the International Agency for Research on Cancer (IARC) in Lyon, France, concluded that there was clear evidence of a relationship between onset of obesity (both early and later) and cancer risk (65).

Short stature (including measures of childhood leg length), a reflection of socioeconomic deprivation in childhood, is associated with an increased risk of CHD and stroke, and to some extent diabetes (10, 15, 28–34). Given that short stature, and specifically short leglength, are particularly sensitive indicators of early socioeconomic deprivation, their association with later disease very likely reflects an association between early undernutrition and infectious disease load (27, 66).

Height serves partly as an indicator of socioeconomic and nutritional status in childhood. As has been seen, poor fetal development and poor growth during childhood have been associated with increased cardio-vascular disease risk in adulthood, as have indicators of unfavourable social circumstances in childhood. Conversely, a high calorie intake in childhood may be related to an increased risk of cancer in later life (64). Height is inversely associated with mortality among men and women from all causes, including coronary heart disease, stroke and respiratory disease (67).

Height has also been used as a proxy for usual childhood energy intake, which is particularly related to body mass and the child's level of activity. However, it is clearly an imperfect proxy because when protein intake is adequate (energy appears to be important in this regard only in the first 3 months of life), genetics will define adult height (36). Protein, particularly animal protein, has been shown to have a selective effect in promoting height growth. It has been suggested that childhood obesity is related to excess protein intake and, of course, overweight or obese children tend to be in the upper percentiles for height. Height has been shown to be related to cancer mortality at several sites, including breast, uterus and colon (36). The risk of stroke is increased by accelerated growth in height during childhood (35). As accelerated growth has been linked to development of hypertension in adult life, this may be the mechanism (plus an association with low socioeconomic status).

There is a higher prevalence of raised blood pressure not only in adults of low socioeconomic status (68–74), but also in children from low socioeconomic backgrounds, although the latter is not always associated with higher blood pressure later in life (*10*). Blood pressure has been found to track from childhood to predict hypertension in adulthood, but with stronger tracking seen in older ages of childhood and in adolescence (*75*).

Higher blood pressure in childhood (in combination with other risk factors) causes target organ and anatomical changes that are associated with cardiovascular risk, including reduction in artery elasticity, increased ventricular size and mass, haemodynamic increase in cardiac output and peripheral resistance (*10, 76, 77*). High blood pressure in children is strongly associated with obesity, in particular central obesity, and clusters and tracks with an adverse serum lipid profile (especially LDL cholesterol) and glucose intolerance (*76, 78, 79*). There may be some ethnic differences, although these often seem to be explained by differences in body mass index. A retrospective mortality follow-up of a survey of family diet and health in the United Kingdom (1937–1939) identified significant associations between childhood energy intake and mortality from cancer (*64*).

The presence and tracking of high blood pressure in children and adolescents occurs against a background of unhealthy lifestyles, including excessive intakes of total and saturated fats, cholesterol and salt, inadequate intakes of potassium, and reduced physical activity, often accompanied by high levels of television viewing (*10*). In adolescents, habitual alcohol and tobacco use contributes to raised blood pressure (*76, 80*).

There are three critical aspects of adolescence that have an impact on chronic diseases: (i) the development of risk factors during this period; (ii) the tracking of risk factors throughout life; and, in terms of prevention, (iii) the development of healthy or unhealthy habits that tend to stay throughout life, for example physical inactivity because of television viewing. In older children and adolescents, habitual alcohol and tobacco use contribute to raised blood pressure and the development of other risk factors in early life, most of which track into adulthood.

The clustering of risk factor variables occurs as early as childhood and adolescence, and is associated with atherosclerosis in young adulthood and thus risk of later cardiovascular disease (*81, 82*). This clustering has been described as the metabolic — or "syndrome X" — clustering of physiological disturbances associated with insulin resistance, including hyperinsulinaemia, impaired glucose tolerance, hypertension, elevated plasma triglyceride and low HDL cholesterol (*83, 84*). Raised serum cholesterol both in middle age and in early life are known to be associated with an increased risk of disease later on. The Johns Hopkins Precursor Study showed that serum cholesterol levels in adolescents and young white males were strongly related to subsequent risk of cardiovascular disease mortality and morbidity (*85*).

Although the risk of obesity does not apparently increase in adults who were overweight at 1 and 3 years old, the risk rises steadily thereafter, regardless of parental weight (86). Tracking has also been reported in China, where overweight children were 2.8 times as likely to become overweight adolescents; conversely, underweight children were 3.6 times as likely to remain underweight as adolescents (87). The study found that parental obesity and underweight, and the child's initial body mass index, dietary fat intake and family income helped predict tracking and changes. However, in a prospective cohort study conducted in the United Kingdom, little tracking from childhood overweight to adulthood obesity was found when using a measure of fatness (percentage body fat for age) that was independent of build (88). The authors also found that only children obese at 13 years of age had an increased risk of obesity as adults, and that there was no excess adult health risk from childhood or adolescent overweight. Interestingly, they found that in the thinnest children, the more obese they became as adults, the greater was their subsequent risk of developing chronic diseases.

The real concern about these early manifestations of chronic disease, besides the fact that they are occurring earlier and earlier, is that once they have developed they tend to track in that individual throughout life. On the more positive side, there is evidence that they can be corrected. Overweight and obesity are, however, notoriously difficult to correct after becoming established, and there is an established risk of overweight during childhood persisting into adolescence and adulthood (89). Recent analyses (90, 91) have shown that the later the weight gain in childhood and adolescence, the greater the persistence. More than 60% of overweight children have at least one additional risk factor for cardiovascular disease, such as raised blood pressure, hyperlipidaemia or hyperinsulinaemia, and more than 20% have two or more risk factors (89).

Habits leading to noncommunicable disease development during adolescence
It seems increasingly likely that there are widespread effects of early diet on later body composition, physiology and cognition (45). Such observations "provide strong support for the recent shift away from defining nutritional needs for prevention of acute deficiency symptoms towards long-term prevention of morbidity and mortality" (45).

Increased birth weight increases the risk of obesity later, but children with low birth weight tend to remain small into adulthood (89, 92). In industrialized countries there have been only modest increases in birth weight so the increased levels of obesity described earlier must reflect environmental changes (89).

The "obesogenic" environment appears to be largely directed at the adolescent market, making healthy choices that much more difficult. At the same time, exercise patterns have changed and considerable parts of the day are spent sitting at school, in a factory, or in front of a television or computer. Raised blood pressure, impaired glucose tolerance and dyslipidaemia are associated in children and adolescents with unhealthy lifestyles, such as diets containing excessive intakes of fats (especially saturated), cholesterol and salt, an inadequate intake of fibre and potassium, a lack of exercise, and increased television viewing (10). Physical inactivity and smoking have been found independently to predict CHD and stroke in later life.

It is increasingly recognized that unhealthy lifestyles do not just appear in adulthood but drive the early development of obesity, dyslipidaemia, high blood pressure, impaired glucose tolerance and associated disease risk. In many countries, perhaps most typified by the United States, changes in family eating patterns, including the increased consumption of fast foods, pre-prepared meals and carbonated drinks, have taken place over the past 30 years (89). At the same time, the amount of physical activity has been greatly reduced both at home and in school, as well as by increasing use of mechanized transport.

4.2.4 *Adulthood*

The three critical questions relating to adulthood were identified as: (i) to what extent do risk factors continue to be important in the development of chronic diseases; (ii) to what extent will modifying such risk factors make a difference to the emergence of disease; and (iii) what is the role of risk factor reduction and modification in secondary prevention and the treatment of those with disease? Reviewing the evidence within the framework of a life-course approach highlights the importance of the adult phase of life, it being both the period during which most chronic diseases are expressed, as well as a critical time for the preventive reduction of risk factors and for increasing effective treatment (93).

The most firmly established associations between cardiovascular disease or diabetes and factors in the lifespan are the ones between those diseases and the major known "adult" risk factors, such as tobacco use, obesity, physical inactivity, cholesterol, high blood pressure and alcohol consumption (94). The factors that have been confirmed to lead to an increased risk of CHD, stroke and diabetes are: high blood pressure for CHD or stroke (95, 96); high cholesterol (diet) for CHD (97, 98), and tobacco use for CHD (99). Other associations are robust and consistent, although they have not necessarily been shown to be reversible (10): obesity and physical inactivity for CHD, diabetes and stroke (*100–102*); and heavy or binge drinking for CHD and stroke (*99, 103*). Most of the studies are from developed countries, but supporting evidence from developing countries is beginning to emerge, for example, from India (*104*).

In developed countries, low socioeconomic status is associated with higher risk of cardiovascular disease and diabetes (*105*). As in the affluent industrialized countries, there appears to be an initial preponderance of cardiovascular disease among the higher socioeconomic groups, for example, as has been found in China (*98*). It is presumed that the disease will progressively shift to the more disadvantaged sectors of society (*10*). There is some evidence that this is already happening, especially among women in low-income groups, for example in Brazil (*106*) and South Africa (*107*), as well as in countries in economic transition such as Morocco (*108*).

Other risk factors are continually being recognized or proposed. These include the role of high levels of homocysteine, the related factor of low folate, and the role of iron (*109*). From a social sciences perspective, Losier (*110*) has suggested that socioeconomic level is less important than a certain stability in the physical and social environment. In other words, an individual's sense of understanding of his or her environment, coupled with control over the course and setting of his or her own life appears to be the most important determinant of health. Marmot (*111*), among others, has demonstrated the impact of the wider environment and societal and individual stress on the development of chronic disease.

4.2.5 *Ageing and older people*

There are three critical aspects relating to chronic diseases in the later part of the life-cycle: (i) most chronic diseases will be manifested in this later stage of life; (ii) there is an absolute benefit for ageing individuals and populations in changing risk factors and adopting health-promoting behaviours such as exercise and healthy diets; and (iii) the need to maximize health by avoiding or delaying preventable disability. Along with the societal and disease transitions, there has been a major demographic shift. Although older people are currently defined as those aged 60 years and above (*112*), this definition of older people has a very different meaning from the middle of the last century, when 60 years of age and above often exceeded the average life expectancy, especially in industrialized countries. It is worth remembering, however, that the majority of elderly people will, in fact, be living in the developing world.

Most chronic diseases are present at this period of life — the result of interactions between multiple disease processes as well as more general losses in physiological functions (*113, 114*). Cardiovascular disease peaks at this period, as does type 2 diabetes and some cancers. The main burden of chronic diseases is observed at this stage of life and, therefore, needs to be addressed.

Changing behaviours in older people

In the 1970s, it was thought that risks were not significantly increased after certain late ages and that there would be no benefit in changing habits, such as dietary habits, after 80 years old (*115*) as there was no epidemiological evidence that changing habits would affect mortality or even health conditions among older people. There was also a feeling that people "earned" some unhealthy behaviours simply because of reaching "old age". Then there was a more active intervention phase, when older people were encouraged to change their diets in ways that were probably overly rigorous for the expected benefit. More recently, older people have been encouraged to eat a healthy diet — as large and as varied as possible while maintaining their weight — and particularly to continue exercise (*113, 116*). Liu et al. (*117*) have reported an observed risk of atherosclerotic disease among older women that was approximately 30% less in women who ate 5–10 servings of fruits and vegetables per day than in those who ate 2–5 servings per day. It seems that, as elderly patients have a higher cardiovascular risk, they are more likely to gain from risk factor modification (*118*).

Although this age group has received relatively little attention as regards primary prevention, the acceleration in decline caused by external factors is generally believed to be reversible at any age (*119*). Interventions aimed at supporting the individual and promoting healthier environments will often lead to increased independence in older age.

4.3 Interactions between early and later factors throughout the life course

Low birth weight, followed by subsequent adult obesity, has been shown to impart a particularly high risk of CHD (*120, 121*), as well as diabetes (*18*). Risk of impaired glucose tolerance has been found to be highest in those who had low birth weight, but who subsequently became obese as adults (*18*). A number of recent studies (*12, 13, 25, 59–61, 120*) have demonstrated that there is an increased risk of adult disease when IUGR is followed by rapid catch-up growth in weight and height. Conversely, there is also fairly consistent evidence of higher risk of CHD, stroke, and probably adult onset diabetes with shorter stature (*122, 123*). Further research is needed to define optimal growth in infancy in terms of prevention of chronic disease. A WHO multicentre growth reference study (*124*) currently under way may serve to generate much needed information on this matter.

4.3.1 *Clustering of risk factors*

Impaired glucose tolerance and an adverse lipid profile are seen as early as childhood and adolescence, where they typically appear clustered together with higher blood pressure and relate strongly to obesity, in particular central obesity (*76, 78, 125, 126*). Raised blood pressure, impaired glucose tolerance and dyslipidaemia also tend to be clustered in children and adolescents with unhealthy lifestyles and diets, such as those with excessive intakes of saturated fats, cholesterol and salt, and inadequate intake of fibre. Lack of exercise and increased television viewing add to the risk (*10*). In older children and adolescents, habitual alcohol and tobacco use also contribute to raised blood pressure and to the development of other risk factors in early adulthood. Many of the same factors continue to act throughout the life course. Such clustering represents an opportunity to address more than one risk at a time. The clustering of health-related behaviours is also a well described phenomenon (*127*).

4.3.2 *Intergenerational effects*

Young girls who grow poorly become stunted women and are more likely to give birth to low-birth-weight babies who are then likely to continue the cycle by being stunted in adulthood, and so on (*128*). Maternal birth size is a significant predictor of a child's birth size after controlling for gestational age, sex of the child, socioeconomic status, and maternal age, height and pre-pregnant weight (*129*). There are clear indications of intergenerational factors in obesity, such as parental obesity, maternal gestational diabetes and maternal birth weight. Low maternal birth weight is associated with higher blood pressure levels in the offspring, independent of the relation between the offspring's own birth weight and blood pressure (*7*). Unhealthy lifestyles can also have a direct effect on the health of the next generation, for example, smoking during pregnancy (*9, 130*).

4.4 Gene–nutrient interactions and genetic susceptibility

There is good evidence that nutrients and physical activity influence gene expression and have shaped the genome over several million years of human evolution. Genes define opportunities for health and susceptibility to disease, while environmental factors determine which susceptible individuals will develop illness. In view of changing socioeconomic conditions in developing countries, such added stress may result in exposure of underlying genetic predisposition to chronic diseases. Gene–nutrient interactions also involve the environment. The dynamics of the relationships are becoming better understood but there is still a long way to go in this area, and also in other aspects, such as disease prevention and control. Studies continue on the role of nutrients in gene expression; for example, researchers are currently trying to understand why omega-3 fatty acids suppress or decrease the mRNA of interleukin, which is elevated in atherosclerosis, arthritis and other autoimmune diseases, whereas the omega-6 fatty acids do not (*131*). Studies on genetic variability to dietary response indicate that specific genotypes raise cholesterol levels more than others. The need for targeted diets for individuals and subgroups to prevent chronic diseases was acknowledged as being part of an overall approach to prevention at the population level. However, the practical implications of this issue

for public health policy have only begun to be addressed. For example, a recent study of the relationship between folate and cardiovascular disease revealed that a common single gene mutation that reduces the activity of an enzyme involved in folate metabolism (MTHFR) is associated with a moderate (20%) increase in serum homocysteine and higher risk of both ischaemic heart disease and deep vein thrombosis (*132*).

Although humans have evolved being able to feed on a variety of foods and to adapt to them, certain genetic adaptations and limitations have occurred in relation to diet. Understanding the evolutionary aspects of diet and its composition might suggest a diet that would be consistent with the diet to which our genes were programmed to respond. However, the early diet was presumably one which gave evolutionary advantage to reproduction in the early part of life, and so may be less indicative of guidance for healthy eating, in terms of lifelong health and prevention of chronic disease after reproduction has been achieved. Because there are genetic variations among individuals, changes in dietary patterns have a differential impact on a genetically heterogeneous population, although populations with a similar evolutionary background have more similar genotypes. While targeted dietary advice for susceptible populations, subgroups or individuals is desirable, it is not feasible at present for the important chronic diseases considered in this report. Most are polygenic in nature and rapidly escalating rates suggest the importance of environmental change rather than change in genetic susceptibility.

4.5 Intervening throughout life

There is a vast volume of scientific evidence highlighting the importance of applying a life-course approach to the prevention and control of chronic disease. The picture is, however, still not complete, and the evidence sometimes contradictory. From the available evidence, it is possible to state the following:

- Unhealthy diets, physical inactivity and smoking are confirmed risk behaviours for chronic diseases.

- The biological risk factors of hypertension, obesity and lipidaemia are firmly established as risk factors for coronary heart disease, stroke and diabetes.

- Nutrients and physical activity influence gene expression and may define susceptibility.

- The major biological and behavioural risk factors emerge and act in early life, and continue to have a negative impact throughout the life course.

- The major biological risk factors can continue to affect the health of the next generation.

- An adequate and appropriate postnatal nutritional environment is important.

- Globally, trends in the prevalence of many risk factors are upwards, especially those for obesity, physical inactivity and, in the developing world particularly, smoking.

- Selected interventions are effective but must extend beyond individual risk factors and continue throughout the life course.

- Some preventive interventions early in the life course offer lifelong benefits.

- Improving diets and increasing levels of physical activity in adults and older people will reduce chronic disease risks for death and disability.

- Secondary prevention through diet and physical activity is a complementary strategy in retarding the progression of existing chronic diseases and decreasing mortality and the disease burden from such diseases.

From the above, it is clear that risk factors must be addressed throughout the life course. As well as preventing chronic diseases, there are clearly many other reasons to improve the quality of life of people throughout their lifespan. The intention of primary prevention interventions is to move the profile of the whole population in a healthier direction. Small changes in risk factors in the majority who are at moderate risk can have an enormous impact in terms of population-attributable risk of death and disability. By preventing disease in large populations, small reductions in blood pressure, blood cholesterol and so on can dramatically reduce health costs. For example, it has been demonstrated that improved lifestyles can reduce the risk of progression to diabetes by a striking 58% over 4 years (*133, 134*). Other population studies have shown that up to 80% of cases of coronary heart disease, and up to 90% of cases of type 2 diabetes, could potentially be avoided through changing lifestyle factors, and about one-third of cancers could be avoided by eating healthily, maintaining normal weight and exercising throughout life (*135–137*).

For interventions to have a lasting effect on the risk factor prevalence and the health of societies, it is also essential to change or modify the environment in which these diseases develop. Changes in dietary patterns, the influence of advertising and the globalization of diets, and widespread reduction in physical activity have generally had negative impacts in terms of risk factors, and presumably also in terms of subsequent disease (*138, 139*). Reversing current trends will require a multifaceted public health policy approach.

While it is important to avoid inappropriately applying nutritional guidelines to populations that may differ genetically from those for whom the dietary and risk data were originally determined, to date the information regarding genes or gene combinations is insufficient to define specific dietary recommendations based on a population distribution of specific genetic polymorphisms. Guidelines should try to ensure that the overall benefit of recommendations to the majority of the population substantially outweighs any potential adverse effects on selected subgroups of the population. For example, population-wide efforts to prevent weight gain may trigger a fear of fatness and, therefore, undernutrition in adolescent girls.

The population nutrient goals recommended by the Joint WHO/FAO Expert Consultation at the present meeting are based on current scientific knowledge and evidence, and are intended to be further adapted and tailored to local or national diets and populations, where diet has evolved to be appropriate for the culture and local environment.

The goals are intended to reverse or reduce the impact of unfavourable dietary changes that have occurred over the past century in the industrialized world and more recently in many developing countries. Present nutrient intake goals also need to take into account the effects of long-term environmental changes, i.e. those that have occurred over time-scales of hundreds of years. For example, the metabolic response to periodic famine and chronic food shortage may no longer represent a selective advantage but instead may increase susceptibility to chronic diseases. An abundant stable food supply is a recent phenomenon; it was not a factor until the advent of the industrial revolution (or the equivalent process in more recently industrialized countries).

A combination of physical activity, food variety and extensive social interaction is the most likely lifestyle profile to optimize health, as reflected in increased longevity and healthy ageing. Some available evidence suggests that, within the time frame of a week, at least 20 and probably as many as 30 biologically distinct types of foods, with the emphasis on plant foods, are required for healthy diets.

The recommendations given in this report consider the wider environment, of which the food supply is a major part (see Chapter 3). The implications of the recommendations would be to increase the consumption of fruits and vegetables, to increase the consumption of fish, and to alter the types of fats and oils, as well as the amount of sugars and starch consumed, especially in developed countries. The current move towards increasing animal protein in diets in countries in economic transition is unlikely to be reversed in those countries where there are increased consumer resources, but is unlikely to be conducive to adult health, at least in terms of preventing chronic diseases.

Finally, what success can be expected by developing and updating the scientific basis for national guidelines? The percentage of British adults complying with national dietary guidelines is discouraging; for example, only 2–4% of the population are currently consuming the recommended level of saturated fat, and 5–25% are achieving the recommended levels of fibre. The figures would not be dissimilar in many other developed countries, where the majority of people are not aware of what exactly the dietary guidelines suggest. In using the updated and evidence-based recommendations in this report, national governments should aim to produce dietary guidelines that are simple, realistic and food-based. There is an increasing need, recognized at all levels, for the wider implications to be specifically addressed; these include the implications for agriculture and fisheries, the role of international trade in a globalized world, the impact on countries dependent on primary produce, the effect of macroeconomic policies, and the need for sustainability. The greatest burden of disease will be in the developing world and, in the transitional and industrialized world, amongst the most disadvantaged socioeconomically.

In conclusion, it may be necessary to have three mutually reinforcing strategies that will have different magnitudes of impact over differing time frames. First, with the greatest and most immediate impact, there is the need to address risk factors in adulthood and, increasingly, among older people. Risk-factor behaviours can be modified in these groups and benefits seen within 3–5 years. With all populations ageing, the sheer numbers and potential cost savings are enormous and realizable. Secondly, societal changes towards health-promoting environments need to be greatly expanded as an integral part of any intervention. Ways to reduce the intake of sugars-sweetened drinks (particularly by children) and of high-energy density foods that are micronutrient poor, as well as efforts to curb cigarette smoking and to increase physical activity will have an impact throughout society. Such changes need the active participation of communities, politicians, health systems, town planners and municipalities, as well as the food and leisure industries. Thirdly, the health environment, in which those who are most at risk grow up, needs to change. This is a more targeted and potentially costly approach, but one that has the potential for cost-effective returns even though they are longer term.

References

1. *Diet, nutrition and the prevention of chronic diseases. Report of a WHO Study Group.* Geneva, World Health Organization, 1990 (WHO Technical Report Series, No. 797).

2. *Diet, physical activity and health.* Geneva, World Health Organization, 2002 (documents A55/16 and A55/16 Corr.1).

3. Barker DJP et al. Weight gain in infancy and death from ischaemic heart disease. *Lancet*, 1989, 2:577–580.

4. Barker DJP et al. Type 2 (non-insulin-dependent) diabetes mellitus, hypertension and hyperlipidaemia (syndrome X): relation to reduced fetal growth. *Diabetologia*, 1993, 36:62–67.

5. Barker DJP et al. Growth in utero and serum cholesterol concentrations in adult life. *British Medical Journal*, 1993, 307:1524–1527.

6. Barker DJP. Fetal origins of coronary heart disease. *British Medical Journal*, 1995, 311:171–174.

7. Barker DJP et al. Growth in utero and blood pressure levels in the next generation. *Journal of Hypertension*, 2000, 18:843–846.

8. Barker DJP et al. Size at birth and resilience to effects of poor living conditions in adult life: longitudinal study. *British Medical Journal*, 2001, 323:1273–1276.

9. *Programming of chronic disease by impaired fetal nutrition: evidence and implications for policy and intervention strategies.* Geneva, World Health Organization, 2002 (documents WHO/NHD/02.3 and WHO/NPH/02.1).

10. Aboderin I et al. *Life course perspectives on coronary heart disease, stroke and diabetes: the evidence and implications for policy and research.* Geneva, World Health Organization, 2002 (document WHO/NMH/NPH/02.1).

11. Godfrey KM, Barker DJ. Fetal nutrition and adult disease. *American Journal of Clinical Nutrition,* 2000, 71(Suppl. 5):S1344–S1352.

12. Forsén T et al. The fetal and childhood growth of persons who develop type II diabetes. *Annals of Internal Medicine*, 2000, 33:176–182.

13. Eriksson JG et al. Catch-up growth in childhood and death from coronary heart disease: a longitudinal study. *British Medical Journal*, 1999, 318:427–431.

14. Forsén T et al. Growth in utero and during childhood in women who develop coronary heart disease: a longitudinal study. *British Medical Journal*, 1999, 319:1403–1407.

15. Rich-Edwards JW et al. Birth weight and the risk of type II diabetes mellitus in adult women. *Annals of Internal Medicine*, 1999, 130:278–284.

16. Leon DA et al. Reduced fetal growth rate and increased risk of death from ischaemic heart disease: cohort study of 15 000 Swedish men and women born 1915–29. *British Medical Journal*, 1998, 317:241–245.

17. McKeigue PM. Diabetes and insulin action. In: Kuh D, Ben-Shlomo Y, eds. *A life course approach to chronic disease epidemiology*. Oxford, Oxford University Press, 1997:78–100.

18. Lithell HO et al. Relation of size at birth to non-insulin dependent diabetes and insulin concentrations in men aged 50–60 years. *British Medical Journal*, 1996, **312**:406–410.

19. Martyn CN, Barker DJP, Osmond C. Mother's pelvic size, fetal growth and death from stroke and coronary heart disease in men in the UK. *Lancet*, 1996, **348**:1264–1268.

20. Martyn CN, Barker DJ. Reduced fetal growth increases risk of cardiovascular disease. *Health Reports*, 1994, **6**:45–53.

21. McCance DR et al. Birthweight and non-insulin dependent diabetes: thrifty genotype, thrifty phenotype or surviving small baby genotype? *British Medical Journal*, 1994, **308**:942–945.

22. Fall CHD et al. Size at birth, maternal weight, and type II diabetes in South India. *Diabetic Medicine*, 1998, **15**:220–227.

23. Valdez R et al. Birthweight and adult health outcomes in a biethnic population in the USA. *Diabetologia*, 1994, **35**:444–446.

24. Kuh D, Ben-Shlomo Y. *A life course approach to chronic disease epidemiology*. Oxford, Oxford University Press, 1997.

25. Eriksson JG et al. Early growth and coronary heart disease in later life: longitudinal study. *British Medical Journal*, 2001, **322**:949–953.

26. Walker SP et al. The effects of birth weight and postnatal linear growth on blood pressure at age 11–12 years. *Journal of Epidemiology and Community Health*, 2001, **55**:394–398.

27. Gunnell DJ et al. Socio-economic and dietary influences on leg length and trunk length in childhood: a reanalysis of the Carnegie (Boyd Orr) survey of diet and health in prewar Britain (1937–39). *Pediatric and Perinatal Epidemiology*, 1998, **12**(Suppl. 1):96–113.

28. McCarron P et al. The relation between adult height and haemorrhagic and ischaemic stroke in the Renfew/Paisley Study. *Journal of Epidemiology and Community Health*, 2001, **55**:404–405.

29. Forsén T et al. Short stature and coronary heart disease: a 35-year follow-up of the Finnish cohorts of the seven countries study. *Journal of Internal Medicine*, 2000, **248**:326–332.

30. Hart CL, Hole DJ, Davey-Smith G. Influence of socioeconomic circumstances in early and later life on stroke risk among men in a Scottish cohort. *Stroke*, 2000, **31**:2093–2097.

31. Jousilahti P et al. Relation of adult height to cause-specific and total mortality: a prospective follow-up study of 31,199 middle-aged men and women. *American Journal of Epidemiology*, 2000, **151**:1112–1120.

32. McCarron P et al. Adult height is inversely associated with ischaemic stroke. The Caerphilly and Speedwell Collaborative Studies. *Journal of Epidemiology and Community Health*, 2000, **54**:239–240.

33. Wannamethee SG et al. Adult height, stroke and coronary heart disease. *American Journal of Epidemiology*, 1998, **148**:1069–1076.

34. **Marmot MG et al**. Contributions of job control and other risk factors to social variations in coronary heart disease incidence. *Lancet*, 1997, **350**:235–239.

35. **Eriksson JG et al**. Early growth, adult income, and risk of stroke. *Stroke*, 2000, **31**:869–874.

36. **Must A, Lipman RD**. Childhood energy intake and cancer mortality in adulthood. *Nutrition Reviews*, 1999, **57**:21–24.

37. **Singhal A, Cole TJ, Lucas A**. Early nutrition in preterm infants and later blood pressure: two cohorts after randomized trials. *Lancet*, 2001, **357**:413–419.

38. **Wilson AC et al**. Relation of infant feeding to adult serum cholesterol concentration and death from ischaemic heart disease. *British Medical Journal*, 1998, **316**:21–25.

39. **Ravelli AC et al**. Infant feeding and adult glucose tolerance, lipid profile, blood pressure, and obesity. *Archives of Disease in Childhood*, 2000, **82**:248–252.

40. **Gillman MW et al**. Risk of overweight among adolescents who were breastfed as infants. *Journal of the American Medical Association*, 2001, **285**:2461–2467.

41. **von Kries R et al**. Does breast-feeding protect against childhood obesity? *Advances in Experimental Medicine and Biology*, 2000, **478**:29–39.

42. **von Kries R et al**. Breast feeding and obesity: cross-sectional study. *British Medical Journal*, 1999, **319**:147–150.

43. **Kramer MS**. Do breast-feeding and delayed introduction of solid foods protect against subsequent obesity? *Journal of Pediatrics*, 1981, **98**:883–887.

44. **Dietz WH**. Breastfeeding may help prevent childhood overweight. *Journal of the American Medical Association*, 2001, **285**:2506–2507.

45. **Roberts SB**. Prevention of hypertension in adulthood by breastfeeding? *Lancet*, 2001, **357**:406–407.

46. **Wingard DL et al**. Is breast-feeding in infancy associated with adult longevity? *American Journal of Public Health*, 1994, **84**:1456–1462.

47. **Fall C**. Nutrition in early life and later outcome. *European Journal of Clinical Nutrition*, 1992, **46**(Suppl. 4):S57–S63.

48. **Davis MK**. Breastfeeding and chronic disease in childhood and adolescence. *Pediatric Clinics of North America*, 2001, **48**:125–141.

49. **Reiser RB et al**. Studies on a possible function for cholesterol in milk. *Nutrition Reports International*, 1979, **19**:835–849.

50. **Mott GE, Lewis DS, McGill HC**. Deferred effects of preweaning nutrition on lipid metabolism. *Annals of the New York Academy of Sciences*, 1991, **623**:70–80.

51. **van Biervliet JP et al**. Plasma apoprotein and lipid patterns in newborns: influence of nutritional factors. *Acta Paediatrica Scandinavica*, 1981, **70**:851–856.

52. **Carlson SE, DeVoe PW, Barness LA**. Effect of infant diets with different polyunsaturated to saturated fat ratios on circulating high density lipoproteins. *Journal of Pediatric Gastroenterology and Nutrition*, 1982, **1**:303–309.

53. **Darmady JM, Fosbrooke AS, Lloyd JK**. Prospective study of serum cholesterol levels during the first year of life. *British Medical Journal*, 1972, **2**:685–688.

54. **Mize CE et al**. Lipoprotein-cholesterol responses in healthy infants fed defined diets from ages 1 to 12 months: comparison of diets predominant in oleic acid

versus linoleic acid, with parallel observations in infants fed a human milk-based diet. *Journal of Lipid Research*, 1995, **36**:1178–1187.

55. **Grundy SM, Denke MA**. Dietary influences on serum lipids and lipoproteins. *Journal of Lipid Research*, 1990, **31**:1149–1172.

56. **Mensink RP, Katan MB**. Effect of dietary fatty acids on serum lipids and lipoproteins. A meta-analysis of 27 trials. *Arteriosclerosis and Thrombosis*, 1992, **12**:911–919.

57. **Arifeen SE et al**. Infant growth patterns in the slums of Dhaka in relation to birth weight, intrauterine growth retardation, and prematurity. *American Journal of Clinical Nutrition*, 2000, **72**:1010–1017.

58. **Bavdekar A et al**. Insulin resistance in 8-year-old Indian children. *Diabetes*, 1999, **48**:2422–2429.

59. **Yajnik CS**. The insulin resistance epidemic in India: fetal origins, later lifestyle, or both? *Nutrition Reviews*, 2001, **59**:1–9.

60. **Yajnik CS**. Interactions of perturbations of intrauterine growth and growth during childhood on the risk of adult-onset disease. *Proceedings of the Nutrition Society*, 2000, **59**:257–265.

61. **Fall CHD et al**. The effects of maternal body composition before pregnancy on fetal growth: the Pune Maternal Nutrition Study. In: O'Brien PMS, Wheeler T, Barker DJP, eds. *Fetal programming influences on development and disease in later life*. London, Royal College of Obstetricians and Gynaecologists Press, 1999:231–245.

62. **Lucas A, Fewtrell MS, Cole TJ**. Fetal origins of adult disease – the hypothesis revisited. *British Medical Journal*, 1999, **319**:245–249.

63. **Must A et al**. Long-term morbidity and mortality of overweight adolescents. A follow-up of the Harvard Growth Study. *New England Journal of Medicine*, 1992, **327**:1350–1355.

64. **Frankel S, Gunnel DJ, Peters TJ**. Childhood energy intake and adult mortality from cancer: the Boyd Orr Cohort Study. *British Medical Journal*, 1998, **316**:499–504.

65. *Weight control and physical activity*. Lyon, International Agency for Research on Cancer, 2002 (IARC Handbooks of Cancer Prevention, Vol. 6).

66. **Davey-Smith G, Shipley M, Leon DA**. Height and mortality from cancer among men: prospective observational study. *British Medical Journal*, 1998, **317**:1351–1352.

67. **Davey-Smith G et al**. Height and risk of death among men and women: aetiological implications of associations with cardiorespiratory disease and cancer mortality. *Journal of Epidemiology and Community Health*, 2000, **54**:97–103.

68. **Bartley M et al**. Social distribution of cardiovascular disease risk factors: change among men 1984–1993. *Journal of Epidemiology and Community Health*, 2000, **54**:806–814.

69. **Manhem K et al**. Social gradients in cardiovascular risk factors and symptoms of Swedish men and women: the Göteborg MONICA Study. *Journal of Cardiovascular Risk*, 2000, **7**:259–318.

70. Colhoun HM, Hemingway H, Poulter N. Socio-economic status and blood pressure: an overview analysis. *Journal of Human Hypertension*, 1998, 12:91–110.

71. Lynch JW et al. Do cardiovascular risk factors explain the relation between socioeconomic status, risk of all-cause mortality, cardiovascular mortality, and acute myocardial infarction? *American Journal of Epidemiology*, 1996, 144:934–942.

72. Myllykangas M et al. Haemostatic and other cardiovascular risk factors, and socioeconomic status among middle-aged Finnish men. *International Journal of Epidemiology*, 1995, **24**:1110–1116.

73. Luepker RV et al. Socioeconomic status and coronary heart disease risk factor trends. The Minnesota Heart Survey. *Circulation*, 1993, **88**:2172–2179.

74. Marmot M. Socioeconomic determinants of CHD mortality. *International Journal of Epidemiology*, 1989, **18**(Suppl. 1):S196–S202.

75. Whincup P, Cook D. Blood pressure and hypertension. In: Kuh D, Ben-Shlomo Y, eds. *A life course approach to chronic disease epidemiology.* Oxford, Oxford University Press, 1997:121–144.

76. Berenson GS et al. *Cardiovascular risk in early life: the Bogalusa Heart Study.* Kalamazoo, MI, The Upjohn Company, 1991 (Current Concepts Series).

77. Bao W et al. Essential hypertension predicted by tracking of elevated blood pressure from childhood to adulthood: the Bogalusa Heart Study. *American Journal of Hypertension*, 1995, **8**:657–665.

78. Tan F et al. Tracking of cardiovascular risk factors and a cohort study on hyperlipidemia in rural schoolchildren in Japan. *Journal of Epidemiology*, 2000, 10:255–261.

79. Tershakovec AM et al. Age-related changes in cardiovascular disease risk factors of hypercholesteraemic children. *Journal of Pediatrics*, 1998, 132:414–420.

80. Okasha M et al. Determinants of adolescent blood pressure: findings from the Glasgow University student cohort. *Journal of Human Hypertension*, 2000, 14:117–124.

81. Bao W et al. Persistence of multiple cardiovascular risk clustering related to Syndrome X from childhood to young adulthood: the Bogalusa Heart Study. *Archives of Internal Medicine*, 1994, **154**:1842–1847.

82. Berenson GS et al. Association between multiple cardiovascular risk factors and atherosclerosis in children and young adults. *New England Journal of Medicine*, 1998, **338**:1650–1656.

83. Reaven GM. Role of insulin resistance in human disease. *Diabetes*, 1988, 37:1595–1607.

84. DeFronzo RA, Ferrannini E. Insulin resistance. A multifaceted syndrome responsible for NIDDM, obesity, hypertension, dyslipidaemia, and athero-sclerotic cardiovascular disease. *Diabetes Care*, 1991, **14**:173–194.

85. Klag MG et al. Serum cholesterol in young men and subsequent cardiovascular disease. *New England Journal of Medicine*, 1993, **328**:313–318.

86. Whitaker RC et al. Predicting obesity in young adulthood from childhood and parental obesity. *New England Journal of Medicine*, 1997, **337**:869–873.

87. Wang Y, Ge K, Popkin BM. Tracking of body mass index from childhood to adolescence: a 6-y follow-up study in China. *American Journal of Clinical Nutrition,* 2000, **72**:1018–1024.

88. Wright CM et al. Implications of childhood obesity for adult health: findings from thousand families cohort study. *British Medical Journal,* 2001, **323**:1280–1284.

89. Dietz WH. The obesity epidemic in young children. *British Medical Journal,* 2001, **322**:313–314.

90. Parsons TJ, Power C, Manor O. Fetal and early life growth and body mass index from birth to early adulthood in a 1958 British cohort: longitudinal study. *British Medical Journal,* 2001, **323**:1331–1335.

91. Parsons TJ et al. Childhood predictors of adult obesity: a systematic review. *International Journal of Obesity and Related Metabolic Disorders,* 1999, **23**(Suppl. 8):S1–S107.

92. Strauss RS. Adult functional outcome of those born small for gestational age: twenty-six-year follow-up of the 1970 British birth cohort. *Journal of the American Medical Association,* 2000, **283**:625–632.

93. Mann JI. Diet and risk of coronary heart disease and type II diabetes. *Lancet,* 2002, **360**:783–789.

94. Elisaf M. The treatment of coronary heart disease: an update. Part 1: an overview of the risk factors for cardiovascular disease. *Current Medical Research and Opinion,* 2001, **17**:18–26.

95. Kannel WB. Blood pressure as a cardiovascular risk factor: prevention and treatment. *Journal of the American Medical Association,* 1996, **275**:1571–1576.

96. MacMahon S et al. Blood pressure, stroke and coronary heart disease. Part 1. Prolonged differences in blood pressure: prospective observational studies corrected for the regression dilution bias. *Lancet,* 1990, **335**:765–774.

97. Hooper L et al. Reduced or modified dietary fat for preventing cardiovascular disease *Cochrane Database of Systematic Reviews,* 2003 (1): CD 002137. (available on the Internet at http://www.update-software.com/cochrane).

98. Hu F et al. Prospective study of major dietary patterns and risk of coronary heart disease in men. *American Journal of Clinical Nutrition,* 2000, **72**:912–921.

99. Lopez A. Alcohol and smoking as risk factors. In: Chamie J, Cliquet L, eds. *Health and mortality: issues of global concern. Proceedings of the Symposium on Health and Mortality, Brussels, 19–22 November 1997.* New York, NY, United Nations Department of Economic and Social Affairs, 1999:374–411.

100. Davey-Smith G et al. Physical activity and cause specific mortality in the Whitehall Study. *Public Health,* 2000, **114**:308–315.

101. Wannamethee SG, Shaper AG, Walker M. Changes in physical activity, mortality and incidence of coronary heart disease in older men. *Lancet,* 1998, **351**:1603–1608.

102. Jousilahti P et al. Body weight, cardiovascular risk factors, and coronary mortality: 15-year follow-up of middle-aged men and women in eastern Finland. *Circulation,* 1996, **93**:1372–1379.

103. Kauhanen J et al. Beer bingeing and mortality. Results from the Kuoipo ischaemic heart disease risk factor study: a prospective population based study. *British Medical Journal,* 1997, **315**:846–851.

104. **Gupta PC, Mehta HC**. Cohort study of all-cause mortality among tobacco users in Mumbai, India. *Bulletin of the World Health Organization*, 2000, **78**:877–883.

105. **Davey-Smith G**. Socioeconomic differentials. In: Kuh D, Ben-Shlomo Y, eds. *A life course approach to chronic disease epidemiology*. Oxford, Oxford University Press, 1997:242–273.

106. **Monteiro CA, Conde WL, Popkin BM**. Is obesity replacing or adding to undernutrition? Evidence from different social classes of Brazil. *Public Health Nutrition*, 2002, **5**:105–112.

107. **Bourne LT, Lambert EV, Steyn K**. Where does the black population of South Africa stand on the nutrition transition? *Public Health Nutrition*, 2002, **5**:157–162.

108. **Benjelloun S**. Nutrition transition in Morocco. *Public Health Nutrition*, 2002, **5**:135–140.

109. **Nelson RL**. Iron and colorectal cancer risk: human studies. *Nutrition Reviews*, 2001, **59**:140–148.

110. **Losier L**. Ambiocontrol as a primary factor of health. *Social Science and Medicine*, 1993, **37**:735–743.

111. **Marmot M**. Aetiology of coronary heart disease. Fetal and infant growth and socioeconomic factors in adult life may act together. *British Medical Journal*, 2001, **323**:1261–1262.

112. *Active ageing: a policy framework*. Geneva, World Health Organization, 2002 (document WHO/NMH/NPH/02.8).

113. **Darnton-Hill I, Coyne ET, Wahlqvist ML**. Assessment of nutritional status. In: Ratnaike R, ed. *A practical guide to geriatric practice*. Sydney, McGraw-Hill, 2001:424–439.

114. **Manton KG, Corder L, Stallard E**. Chronic disability trends in elderly United States populations: 1982–1994. *Proceedings of the National Academy of Sciences of the United States of America*, 1997, **94**:2593–2598.

115. **Lasheras C, Fernandez S, Patterson AM**. Mediterranean diet and age with respect to overall survival in institutionalised, non-smoking elderly people. *American Journal of Clinical Nutrition*, 2000, **71**:987–992.

116. **World Health Organization/Tufts University School of Nutrition Science and Policy**. *Keep fit for life: meeting the nutritional needs of older persons*. Geneva, World Health Organization, 2002.

117. **Liu S et al**. Fruit and vegetable intake and risk of cardiovascular disease: the Women's Health Study. *American Journal of Clinical Nutrition*, 2000, **72**:922–928.

118. **Smith GD, Song F, Sheldon TA**. Cholesterol lowering and mortality: the importance of considering initial level of risk. *British Medical Journal*, 1993, **306**:1367–1373.

119. *Ageing: exploding the myths*. Geneva, World Health Organization, 1999 (document WHO/HSL/AHE/99.1).

120. **Yajnik CS**. The lifecycle effects of nutrition and body size on adult obesity, diabetes and cardiovascular disease. *Obesity Reviews*, 2002, **3**:217–224.

121. **Frankel S et al**. Birthweight, body mass index in middle age and incident coronary heart disease. *Lancet*, 1996, **348**:1478–1480.

122. **Eriksson J et al**. Fetal and childhood growth and hypertension in adult life. *Hypertension*, 2000, **36**:790–794.

123. Leon DA et al. Failure to realise growth potential in utero and adult obesity in relation to blood pressure in 50-year-old Swedish men. *British Medical Journal*, 1996, **312**:401–406.

124. Garza C, de Onis M. A new international growth reference for young children. *American Journal of Clinical Nutrition*, 1999, **70**(Suppl.):S169–S172.

125. Twisk JW et al. Clustering of biological risk factors for cardiovascular disease and the longitudinal relationship with lifestyle of an adolescent population: the Northern Ireland Young Hearts Project. *Journal of Cardiovascular Risk*, 1999, **6**:355–362.

126. Raitakari OT et al. Clustering of risk factors for coronary heart disease in children and adolescents. The Cardiovascular Risk in Young Finns Study. *Acta Paediatrica*, 1994, **83**:935–940.

127. Koo LC et al. Dietary and lifestyle correlates of passive smoking in Hong Kong, Japan, Sweden, and the USA. *Social Science and Medicine*, 1997, **45**:159–169.

128. United Nations Children's Fund. *The state of the world's children 1998*. Oxford and New York, Oxford University Press, 1998.

129. Ramakrishnan U et al. Role of intergenerational effects on linear growth. *Journal of Nutrition*, 1999, **129**(Suppl. 2):S544–S549.

130. Montgomery SM, Ekbom A. Smoking during pregnancy and diabetes mellitus in a British longitudinal birth cohort. *British Medical Journal*, 2002, **324**:26–27.

131. Simopoulos AP, Pavlow KN, eds. *Nutrition and fitness: diet, genes, physical activity and health. Proceedings of 4th International Conference on Nutrition and Fitness, Athens, May 2000*. New York, NY, Karger, 2001 (World Review of Nutrition and Dietetics, Vol. 89).

132. Wald DS, Law M, Morris JK. Homocysteine and cardiovascular disease: evidence on causality from a meta-analysis. *British Medical Journal, 2002*, 325:1202–1208.

133. Diabetes Prevention Program Research Group. Reduction in the incidence of type II diabetes with lifestyle intervention or metformin. *New England Journal of Medicine*, 2002, **346**:343–403.

134. Tuomilehto J et al. Prevention of type II diabetes mellitus by changes in lifestyle among subjects with impaired glucose tolerance. *New England Journal of Medicine*, 2001, **344**:1343–1350.

135. Stampfer MJ et al. Primary prevention of coronary heart disease in women through diet and lifestyle. *New England Journal of Medicine*, 2000, **343**:16–22.

136. Hu FB et al. Diet, lifestyle, and the risk of type II diabetes mellitus in women. *New England Journal of Medicine*, 2001, **345**:790–797.

137. Key TJ. The effect of diet on risk of cancer. *Lancet*, 2002, **360**:861–868.

138. *Globalization, diets and noncommunicable diseases*. Geneva, World Health Organization, 2002.

139. Beaglehole R, Yach D. Globalization and the prevention and control of noncommunicable disease: the neglected chronic diseases of adults. *Lancet* (in press).

5. Population nutrient intake goals for preventing diet-related chronic diseases

5.1 Overall goals

5.1.1 *Background*

Population nutrient intake goals represent the population average intake that is judged to be consistent with the maintenance of health in a population. Health, in this context, is marked by a low prevalence of diet-related diseases in the population.

Seldom is there a single "best value" for such a goal. Instead, consistent with the concept of a safe range of nutrient intakes for individuals, there is often a range of population averages that would be consistent with the maintenance of health. If existing population averages fall outside this range, or trends in intake suggest that the population average will move outside the range, health concerns are likely to arise. Sometimes there is no lower limit; this implies that there is no evidence that the nutrient is required in the diet and hence low intakes should not give rise to concern. It would be of concern if a large proportion of values were outside the defined goals.

5.1.2 *Strength of evidence*

Ideally the definition of an increased or a decreased risk should be based on a relationship that has been established by multiple randomized controlled trials of interventions on populations that are representative of the target of a recommendation, but this type of evidence is often not available. The recommended dietary/nutrition practice should modify the attributable risk of the undesirable exposure in that population.

The following criteria are used to describe the strength of evidence in this report. They are based on the criteria used by the World Cancer Research Fund (*1*), but have been modified by the Expert Consultation to include the results of controlled trials where relevant and available. In addition, consistent evidence on community and environmental factors which lead to behaviour changes and thereby modify risks has been taken into account in categorizing risks. This applies particularly to the complex interaction between environmental factors that affect excess weight gain, a risk factor which the Consultation recognized as contributing to many of the problems being considered.

- *Convincing evidence*. Evidence based on epidemiological studies showing consistent associations between exposure and disease, with little or no evidence to the contrary. The available evidence is based on a substantial number of studies including prospective observational studies and where relevant, randomized controlled trials of sufficient size, duration and quality showing consistent effects. The association should be biologically plausible.

- *Probable evidence.* Evidence based on epidemiological studies showing fairly consistent associations between exposure and disease, but where there are perceived shortcomings in the available evidence or some evidence to the contrary, which precludes a more definite judgement. Shortcomings in the evidence may be any of the following: insufficient duration of trials (or studies); insufficient trials (or studies) available; inadequate sample sizes; incomplete follow-up. Laboratory evidence is usually supportive. Again, the association should be biologically plausible.

- *Possible evidence.* Evidence based mainly on findings from case–control and cross-sectional studies. Insufficient randomized controlled trials, observational studies or non-randomized controlled trials are available. Evidence based on non-epidemiological studies, such as clinical and laboratory investigations, is supportive. More trials are required to support the tentative associations, which should also be biologically plausible.

- *Insufficient evidence.* Evidence based on findings of a few studies which are suggestive, but are insufficient to establish an association between exposure and disease. Limited or no evidence is available from randomized controlled trials. More well designed research is required to support the tentative associations.

The strength of evidence linking dietary and lifestyle factors to the risk of developing obesity, type 2 diabetes, CVD, cancer, dental diseases, osteoporosis, graded according to the above categories, is summarized in tabular form, and attached to this report as an Annex.

5.1.3 *A summary of population nutrient intake goals*

The population nutrient intake goals for consideration by national and regional bodies establishing dietary recommendations for the prevention of diet-related chronic diseases are presented in Table 6. These recommendations are expressed in numerical terms, rather than as increases or decreases in intakes of specific nutrients, because the desirable change will depend upon existing intakes in the particular population, and could be in either direction.

In Table 6, attention is directed towards the energy-supplying macronutrients. This must not be taken to imply a lack of concern for the other nutrients. Rather, it is a recognition of the fact that previous reports issued by FAO and WHO have provided limited guidance on the meaning of a "balanced diet" described in terms of the proportions of the various energy sources, and that there is an apparent consensus on this aspect of diet in relation to effects on the chronic non-deficiency diseases.

This report therefore complements these existing reports on energy and nutrient requirements issued by FAO and WHO (2–4). In translating these goals into dietary guidelines, due consideration should be given to the process for setting up national dietary guidelines (5).

Table 6
Ranges of population nutrient intake goals

Dietary factor	Goal (% of total energy, unless otherwise stated)
Total fat	15–30%
Saturated fatty acids	<10%
Polyunsaturated fatty acids (PUFAs)	6–10%
n-6 Polyunsaturated fatty acids (PUFAs)	5–8%
n-3 Polyunsaturated fatty acids (PUFAs)	1–2%
Trans fatty acids	<1%
Monounsaturated fatty acids (MUFAs)	By difference[a]
Total carbohydrate	55–75%[b]
Free sugars[c]	<10%
Protein	10–15%[d]
Cholesterol	<300 mg per day
Sodium chloride (sodium)[e]	<5 g per day (<2 g per day)
Fruits and vegetables	⩾400 g per day
Total dietary fibre	From foods[f]
Non-starch polysaccharides (NSP)	From foods[f]

[a] This is calculated as: total fat – (saturated fatty acids + polyunsaturated fatty acids + trans fatty acids).
[b] The percentage of total energy available after taking into account that consumed as protein and fat, hence the wide range.
[c] The term "free sugars" refers to all monosaccharides and disaccharides added to foods by the manufacturer, cook or consumer, plus sugars naturally present in honey, syrups and fruit juices.
[d] The suggested range should be seen in the light of the Joint WHO/FAO/UNU Expert Consultation on Protein and Amino Acid Requirements in Human Nutrition, held in Geneva from 9 to 16 April 2002 (2).
[e] Salt should be iodized appropriately (6). The need to adjust salt iodization, depending on observed sodium intake and surveillance of iodine status of the population, should be recognized.
[f] See page 58, under "Non-starch polysaccharides".

Total fat

The recommendations for total fat are formulated to include countries where the usual fat intake is typically above 30% as well as those where the usual intake may be very low, for example less than 15%. Total fat energy of at least 20% is consistent with good health. Highly active groups with diets rich in vegetables, legumes, fruits and wholegrain cereals may, however, sustain a total fat intake of up to 35% without the risk of unhealthy weight gain.

For countries where the usual fat intake is between 15% and 20% of energy, there is no direct evidence for men that raising fat intake to 20% will be beneficial (7, 8). For women of reproductive age at least 20% has been recommended by the Joint FAO/WHO Expert Consultation on Fats and Oils in Human Nutrition that met in 1993 (3).

Free sugars

It is recognized that higher intakes of free sugars threaten the nutrient quality of diets by providing significant energy without specific nutrients. The Consultation considered that restriction of free sugars was also likely to contribute to reducing the risk of unhealthy weight gain, noting that:

- Free sugars contribute to the overall energy density of diets.
- Free sugars promote a positive energy balance. Acute and short-term studies in human volunteers have demonstrated increased total energy intake when the energy density of the diet is increased, whether by free sugars or fat (9–11). Diets that are limited in free sugars have been shown to reduce total energy intake and induce weight loss (12, 13).
- Drinks that are rich in free sugars increase overall energy intake by reducing appetite control. There is thus less of a compensatory reduction of food intake after the consumption of high-sugars drinks than when additional foods of equivalent energy content are provided (11, 14–16). A recent randomized trial showed that when soft drinks rich in free sugars are consumed there is a higher energy intake and a progressive increase in body weight when compared with energy-free drinks that are artificially sweetened (17). Children with a high consumption of soft drinks rich in free sugars are more likely to be overweight and to gain excess weight (16).

The Consultation recognized that a population goal for free sugars of less than 10% of total energy is controversial. However, the Consultation considered that the studies showing no effect of free sugars on excess weight have limitations. The CARMEN study (Carbohydrate Ratio Management in European National diets) was a multicentre, randomized trial that tested the effects on body weight and blood lipids in overweight individuals of altering the ratio of fat to carbohydrate, as well as the ratio of simple to complex carbohydrate per se. A greater weight reduction was observed with the high complex carbohydrate diet relative to the simple carbohydrate one; the difference, however was not statistically significant (18). Nevertheless, an analysis of weight change and metabolic indices for those with metabolic syndrome revealed a clear benefit of replacing simple by complex carbohydrates (19). The Consultation also examined the results of studies that found an inverse relationship between free sugars intakes and total fat intake. Many of these studies are methodologically inappropriate for determining the causes of excess weight gain, since the percentage of calories from fat will decrease as the percentage of calories from carbohydrates increases and vice versa. Furthermore, these analyses do not usually distinguish between free sugars in foods and free sugars in drinks. Thus, these analyses are not good predictors of the responses in energy intake to a selective reduction in free sugars intake.

Non-starch polysaccharides (NSP)

Wholegrain cereals, fruits and vegetables are the preferred sources of non-starch polysaccharides (NSP). The best definition of dietary fibre remains to be established, given the potential health benefits of resistant starch. The recommended intake of fruits and vegetables (see below) and consumption of wholegrain foods is likely to provide > 20 g per day of NSP (> 25 g per day of total dietary fibre).

Fruits and vegetables

The benefit of fruits and vegetables cannot be ascribed to a single or mix of nutrients and bioactive substances. Therefore, this food category was included rather than the nutrients themselves. The category of tubers (i.e. potatoes, cassava) should not be included in fruits and vegetables.

Body mass index (BMI)

The goal for body mass index (BMI) included in this report follows the recommendations made by the WHO Expert Consultation on Obesity that met in 1997 (20). At the population level, the goal is for an adult median BMI of 21–23 kg/m². For individuals, the recommendation is to maintain a BMI in the range 18.5–24.9 kg/ m² and to avoid a weight gain greater than 5 kg during adult life.

Physical activity

The goal for physical activity focuses on maintaining healthy body weight. The recommendation is for a total of one hour per day on most days of the week of moderate-intensity activity, such as walking. This level of physical activity is needed to maintain a healthy body weight, particularly for people with sedentary occupations. The recommendation is based on calculations of energy balance and on an analysis of the extensive literature on the relationships between body weight and physical activity. This recommendation is also presented elsewhere (21). Obviously, this quantitative goal cannot be considered as a single "best value" by analogy with the nutrient intake goals. Furthermore, it differs from the following widely accepted public health recommendation (22):

> For better health, people of all ages should include a minimum of 30 minutes of physical activity of moderate intensity (such as brisk walking) on most, if not all, days of the week. For most people greater health benefits can be obtained by engaging in physical activity of more vigorous intensity or of longer duration. This cardio respiratory endurance activity should be supplemented with

strength-developing exercises at least twice a week for adults in order to improve musculo skeletal health, maintain independence in performing the activities of daily life and reduce the risk of falling.

The difference between the two recommendations results from the difference in their focus. A recent symposium on the dose–response relationships between physical activity and health outcomes found evidence that 30 minutes of moderate activity is sufficient for cardiovascular/metabolic health, but not for all health benefits. Because prevention of obesity is a central health goal, the recommendation of 60 minutes a day of moderate-intensity activity is considered appropriate. Activity of moderate intensity is found to be sufficient to have a preventive effect on most, if not all, cardiovascular and metabolic diseases considered in this report. Higher intensity activity has a greater effect on some, although not all, health outcomes, but is beyond the capacity and motivation of a large majority of the population.

Both recommendations include the idea that the daily activity can be accomplished in several short bouts. It is important to point out that both recommendations apply to people who are otherwise sedentary. Some occupational activities and household chores constitute sufficient daily physical exercise.

In recommending physical activity, potential individual risks as well as benefits need to be assessed. In many regions of the world, especially but not exclusively in rural areas of developing countries, an appreciable proportion of the population is still engaged in physically demanding activities relating to agricultural practices and domestic tasks performed without mechanization or with rudimentary tools. Even children may be required to undertake physically demanding tasks at very young ages, such as collecting water and firewood and caring for livestock. Similarly, the inhabitants of poor urban areas may still be required to walk long distances to their jobs, which are usually of a manual nature and often require a high expenditure of energy. Clearly, the recommendation for extra physical activity is not relevant for these sectors of the population.

References

1. World Cancer Research Fund. *Food, nutrition and the prevention of cancer: a global perspective.* Washington, DC, American Institute for Cancer Research, 1997.

2. *Protein and amino acid requirements in human nutrition. Report of a Joint WHO/FAO/ UNU Expert Consultation.* Geneva, World Health Organization, 2003 (in press).

3. *Fats and oils in human nutrition. Report of a Joint FAO/WHO Expert Consultation.* Rome, Food and Agriculture Organization of the United Nations, 1994 (FAO Food and Nutrition Paper, No. 57).

4. *Carbohydrates in human nutrition. Report of a Joint FAO/WHO Expert Consultation.* Rome, Food and Agriculture Organization of the United Nations, 1998 (FAO Food and Nutrition Paper, No. 66).

5. Preparation and use of *food-based dietary guidelines. Report of a Joint FAO/ WHO Consultation*. Geneva, World Health Organization, 1998 (WHO Technical Report Series, No. 880).

6. WHO/UNICEF/ICCIDD. *Recommended iodine levels in salt and guidelines for monitoring their adequacy and effectiveness*. Geneva, World Health Organization, 1996 (document WHO/NUT/96.13).

7. Campbell TC, Parpia B, Chen J. Diet, lifestyle, and the etiology of coronary artery disease: the Cornell China study. *American Journal of Cardiology*, 1998, **82**:18T–21T.

8. Campbell TC, Junshi C. Diet and chronic degenerative diseases: perspectives from China. *American Journal of Clinical Nutrition*, **59**(Suppl. 5):S1153–S1161.

9. Stubbs J, Ferres S, Horgan G. Energy density of foods: effects on energy intake. *Critical Reviews in Food Science and Nutrition*, 2000, **40**:481–515.

10. Rolls BJ, Bell EA. Dietary approaches to the treatment of obesity. *Medical Clinics of North America*, 2000, **84**:401–418.

11. Rolls BJ. Fat and sugar substitutes and the control of food intake. *Annals of the New York Academy of Sciences*, 1997, **819**:180–193.

12. Mann JI et al. Effects on serum-lipids in normal men of reducing dietary sucrose or starch for five months. *Lancet*, 1970, 1:870–872.

13. Smith JB, Niven BE, Mann JI. The effect of reduced extrinsic sucrose intake on plasma triglyceride levels. *European Journal of Clinical Nutrition*, 1996, **50**:498–504.

14. Ludwig DS. The glycemic index: physiological mechanisms relating to obesity, diabetes, and cardiovascular disease. *Journal of American Medical Association*, 2002, **287**:2414–2423.

15. Ebbeling CB, Ludwig DS. Treating obesity in youth: should dietary glycemic load be a consideration? *Advances in Pediatrics*, 2001, **48**:179–212.

16. Ludwig DS, Peterson KE, Gormakaer SL. Relation between consumption of sugar-sweetened drinks and childhood obesity: a prospective, observational analysis. *Lancet*, 2001, **357**:505–508.

17. Raben A et al. Sucrose compared with artificial sweeteners: different effects on ad libitum food intake and body weight after 10 wk of supplementation in overweight subjects. *American Journal of Clinical Nutrition*, 2002, **76**:721–729.

18. Saris WH et al. Randomized controlled trial of changes in dietary carbohydrate/ fat ratio and simple vs complex carbohydrates on body weight and blood lipids: the CARMEN study. The Carbohydrate Ratio Management in European National diets. *International Journal of Obesity and Related Metabolic Disorders*, 2000, **24**:1310–1318.

19. Poppitt SD et al. Long-term effects of ad libitum low-fat, high-carbohydrate diets on body weight and serum lipids in overweight subjects with metabolic syndrome. *American Journal of Clinical Nutrition*, 2002, **75**:11–20.

20. *Obesity: preventing and managing the global epidemic. Report of a WHO Consultation*. Geneva, World Health Organization, 2000 (WHO Technical Report Series, No. 894).

21. *Weight control and physical activity*. Lyon, International Agency for Research on Cancer, 2002 (IARC Handbooks of Cancer Prevention, Vol. 6).

22. *Physical activity and health: a report of the Surgeon General*. Atlanta, GA, US Department of Health and Human Services, Centers for Disease Control and Prevention, National Center for Chronic Disease Prevention and Health Promotion, 1996.

5.2 Recommendations for preventing excess weight gain and obesity

5.2.1 *Background*

Almost all countries (high-income and low-income alike) are experiencing an obesity epidemic, although with great variation between and within countries. In low-income countries, obesity is more common in middle-aged women, people of higher socioeconomic status and those living in urban communities. In more affluent countries, obesity is not only common in the middle-aged, but is becoming increasingly prevalent among younger adults and children. Furthermore, it tends to be associated with lower socioeconomic status, especially in women, and the urban–rural differences are diminished or even reversed.

It has been estimated that the direct costs of obesity accounted for 6.8% (or US$ 70 billion) of total health care costs, and physical inactivity for a further US$ 24 billion, in the United States in 1995. Although direct costs in other industrialized countries are slightly lower, they still consume a sizeable proportion of national health budgets (1). Indirect costs, which are far greater than direct costs, include workdays lost, physician visits, disability pensions and premature mortality. Intangible costs such as impaired quality of life are also enormous. Because the risks of diabetes, cardiovascular disease and hypertension rise continuously with increasing weight, there is much overlap between the prevention of obesity and the prevention of a variety of chronic diseases, especially type 2 diabetes. Population education strategies will need a solid base of policy and environment-based changes to be effective in eventually reversing these trends.

5.2.2 *Trends*

The increasing industrialization, urbanization and mechanization occurring in most countries around the world is associated with changes in diet and behaviour, in particular, diets are becoming richer in high-fat, high energy foods and lifestyles more sedentary. In many developing countries undergoing economic transition, rising levels of obesity often coexist in the same population (or even the same household) with chronic undernutrition. Increases in obesity over the past 30 years have been paralleled by a dramatic rise in the prevalence of diabetes (2).

5.2.3 *Diet, physical activity and excess weight gain and obesity*

Mortality rates increase with increasing degrees of overweight, as measured by BMI. As BMI increases, so too does the proportion of people with one or more comorbid conditions. In one study in the USA (3), over half (53%) of all deaths in women with a BMI > 29 kg/m^2 could be directly attributed to their obesity. Eating behaviours that have been linked to overweight and obesity include snacking/eating frequency, binge-eating patterns, eating out, and (protectively) exclusive breast-feeding. Nutrient factors under investigation include fat, carbohydrate type (including refined carbohydrates such as sugar), the glycaemic index of foods, and fibre. Environmental issues are clearly important, especially as many environments become increasingly "obesogenic" (obesity-promoting).

Physical activity is an important determinant of body weight. In addition, physical activity and physical fitness (which relates to the ability to perform physical activity) are important modifiers of mortality and morbidity related to overweight and obesity. There is firm evidence that moderate to high fitness levels provide a substantially reduced risk of cardiovascular disease and all-cause mortality and that these benefits apply to all BMI levels. Furthermore, high fitness protects against mortality at all BMI levels in men with diabetes. Low cardiovascular fitness is a serious and common comorbidity of obesity, and a sizeable proportion of deaths in overweight and obese populations are probably a result of low levels of cardio-respiratory fitness rather than obesity per se. Fitness is, in turn, influenced strongly by physical activity in addition to genetic factors. These relationships emphasize the role of physical activity in the prevention of overweight and obesity, independently of the effects of physical activity on body weight.

The potential etiological factors related to unhealthy weight gain are listed in Table 7.

5.2.4 *Strength of evidence*

Convincing etiological factors

Regular physical activity (protective) and sedentary lifestyles (causative). There is convincing evidence that regular physical activity is protective against unhealthy weight gain whereas sedentary lifestyles, particularly sedentary occupations and inactive recreation such as watching television, promote it. Most epidemiological studies show smaller risk of weight gain, overweight and obesity among persons who *currently* engage regularly in moderate to large amounts of physical activity (*4*). Studies measuring physical activity at baseline and randomized trials of exercise programmes show more mixed results, probably because of the low adherence to long-term changes. Therefore, it is ongoing physical activity itself rather than previous physical activity or enrolment in an exercise programme that is protective against unhealthy weight gain. The recommendation for individuals to accumulate at least 30 minutes of moderate-intensity physical activity on most days is largely aimed at reducing cardiovascular diseases and overall mortality. The amount needed to prevent unhealthy weight gain is uncertain but is probably significantly greater than this. Preventing weight gain after substantial weight loss probably requires about 60–90 minutes per day. Two meetings recommended by consensus that about 45–60 minutes of moderate-intensity physical activity is needed on most days or every day to prevent unhealthy weight gain (5, 6). Studies aimed at reducing sedentary behaviours have focused primarily on reducing television viewing in children. Reducing viewing times by about 30 minutes a day in children in the United States appears feasible and is associated with reductions in BMI.

Table 7
Summary of strength of evidence on factors that might promote or protect against weight gain and obesity[a]

Evidence	Decreased risk	No relationship	Increased risk
Convincing	Regular physical activity High dietary intake of NSP (dietary fibre)[b]		Sedentary lifestyles High intake of energy-dense micronutrient-poor foods[c]
Probable	Home and school environments that support healthy food choices for children[d] Breastfeeding		Heavy marketing of energy-dense foods[d] and fast-food outlets[d] High intake of sugars-sweetened soft drinks and fruit juices Adverse socioeconomic conditions[d] (in developed countries, especially for women)
Possible	Low glycaemic index foods	Protein content of the diet	Large portion sizes High proportion of food prepared outside the home (developed countries) "Rigid restraint/periodic disinhibition" eating patterns
Insufficient	Increased eating frequency		Alcohol

[a] Strength of evidence: the totality of the evidence was taken into account. The World Cancer Research Fund schema was taken as the starting point but was modified in the following manner: randomized controlled trials were given prominence as the highest ranking study design (randomized controlled trials were not a major source of cancer evidence); associated evidence and expert opinion was also taken into account in relation to environmental determinants (direct trials were usually not available).
[b] Specific amounts will depend on the analytical methodologies used to measure fibre.
[c] Energy-dense and micronutrient-poor foods tend to be processed foods that are high in fat and/or sugars. Low energy-dense (or energy-dilute) foods, such as fruit, legumes, vegetables and whole grain cereals, are high in dietary fibre and water.
[d] Associated evidence and expert opinion included.

A high dietary intake of non-starch polysaccharides (NSP)/dietary fibre (protective). The nomenclature and definitions of NSP (dietary fibre) have changed with time, and many of the available studies used previous definitions, such as soluble and insoluble fibre. Nevertheless, two recent reviews of randomized trials have concluded that the majority of studies show that a high intake of NSP (dietary fibre) promotes weight loss.

Pereira & Ludwig (7) found that 12 out of 19 trials showed beneficial objective effects (including weight loss). In their review of 11 studies of more than 4 weeks duration, involving ad libitum eating Howarth Saltzman & Roberts (8) reported a mean weight loss of 1.9 kg over 3.8 months. There were no differences between fibre type or between fibre consumed in food or as supplements.

High intake of energy-dense micronutrient-poor foods (causative).
There is convincing evidence that a high intake of energy-dense foods promotes weight gain. In high-income countries (and increasingly in low-income countries) these energy-dense foods are not only highly processed (low NSP) but also micronutrient-poor, further diminishing their nutritional value. Energy-dense foods tend to be high in fat (e.g. butter, oils, fried foods), sugars or starch, while energy-dilute foods have a high water content (e.g. fruits and vegetables). Several trials have covertly manipulated the fat content and the energy density of diets, the results of which support the view that so-called "passive over consumption" of total energy occurs when the energy density of the diet is high and that this is almost always the case in high-fat diets. A meta-analysis of 16 trials of ad libitum high-fat versus low-fat diets of at least 2 months duration suggested that a reduction in fat content by 10% corresponds to about a 1 MJ reduction in energy intake and about 3 kg in body weight (9). At a population level, 3 kg equates to about one BMI unit or about a 5% difference in obesity prevalence. However, it is difficult to blind such studies and other non-physiological effects may influence these findings (10). While energy from fat is no more fattening than the same amount of energy from carbohydrate or protein, diets that are high in fat tend to be energy-dense. An important exception to this is diets based predominantly on energy-dilute foods (e.g. vegetables, legumes, fruits) but which have a reasonably high percentage of energy as fat from added oils.

The effectiveness over the long term of most dietary strategies for weight loss, including low-fat diets, remains uncertain unless accompanied by changes in behaviour affecting physical activity and food habits. These latter changes at a public health level require an environment supportive of healthy food choices and an active life. High quality trials to address these issues are urgently needed. A variety of popular weight-loss diets that restrict food choices may result in reduced energy intake and short-term weight loss in individuals but most do not have trial evidence of long-term effectiveness and nutritional adequacy and therefore cannot be recommended for populations.

Probable etiological factors
Home and school environments that promote healthy food and activity choices for children (protective). Despite the obvious importance of the

roles that parents and home environments play on children's eating and physical activity behaviours, there is very little hard evidence available to support this view. It appears that access and exposure to a range of fruits and vegetables in the home is important for the development of preferences for these foods and that parental knowledge, attitudes and behaviours related to healthy diet and physical activity are important in creating role models (*11*). More data are available on the impact of the school environment on nutrition knowledge, on eating patterns and physical activity at school, and on sedentary behaviours at home. Some studies (*12*), but not all, have shown an effect of school-based interventions on obesity prevention. While more research is clearly needed to increase the evidence base in both these areas, supportive home and school environments were rated as a probable etiological influence on obesity.

Heavy marketing of fast-food outlets and energy-dense, micronutrient-poor foods and beverages (causative). Part of the consistent, strong relationships between television viewing and obesity in children may relate to the food advertising to which they are exposed (*13–15*). Fast-food restaurants, and foods and beverages that are usually classified under the "eat least" category in dietary guidelines are among the most heavily marketed products, especially on television. Young children are often the target group for the advertising of these products because they have a significant influence on the foods bought by parents (*16*). The huge expenditure on marketing fast-foods and other "eat least" choices (US$ 11 billion in the United States alone in 1997) was considered to be a key factor in the increased consumption of food prepared outside the home in general and of energy-dense, micronutrient-poor foods in particular. Young children are unable to distinguish programme content from the persuasive intent of advertisements. The evidence that the heavy marketing of these foods and beverages to young children causes obesity is not unequivocal. Nevertheless, the Consultation considered that there is sufficient indirect evidence to warrant this practice being placed in the "probable" category and thus becoming a potential target for interventions (*15–18*).

A high intake of sugars-sweetened beverages (causative). Diets that are proportionally low in fat will be proportionally higher in carbohydrate (including a variable amount of sugars) and are associated with protection against unhealthy weight gain, although a high intake of free sugars in beverages probably promotes weight gain. The physiological effects of energy intake on satiation and satiety appear to be quite different for energy in solid foods as opposed to energy in fluids. Possibly because of reduced gastric distension and faster transit times, the energy contained in fluids is less well "detected" by the body and subsequent food intake is poorly adjusted to account for the energy taken in through beverages (*19*). This is supported by data from cross-sectional, longitudinal, and cross-over studies (*20–22*). The high and increasing consumption of sugars-sweetened drinks by children in many countries is of serious concern. It has been estimated that each additional can or glass of sugars-sweetened drink that they consume every day increases the risk of becoming obese by 60% (*19*). Most of the evidence relates to soda drinks but many fruit drinks and cordials are equally energy-dense and may promote weight gain if drunk in large quantities. Overall, the evidence implicating a high intake of sugars-sweetened drinks in promoting weight gain was considered moderately strong.

Adverse socioeconomic conditions, especially for women in high-income countries (causative). Classically the pattern of the progression of obesity through a population starts with middle-aged women in high-income groups but as the epidemic progresses, obesity becomes more common in people (especially women) in lower socioeconomic status groups. The relationship may even be bi-directional, setting up a vicious cycle (i.e. lower socioeconomic status promotes obesity, and obese people are more likely to end up in groups with low socioeconomic status). The mechanisms by which socioeconomic status influences food and activity patterns are probably multiple and need elucidation. However, people living in circumstances of low socioeconomic status may be more at the mercy of the obesogenic environment because their eating and activity behaviours are more likely to be the "default choices" on offer. The evidence for an effect of low socioeconomic status on predisposing people to obesity is consistent (in higher income countries) across a number of cross-sectional and longitudinal studies (*23*), and was thus rated as a "probable" cause of increased risk of obesity.

Breastfeeding (protective). Breastfeeding as a protective factor against weight gain has been examined in at least 20 studies involving nearly 40 000 subjects. Five studies (including the two largest) found a protective effect, two found that breastfeeding predicted obesity, and the remainder found no relationships. There are probably multiple effects of confounding in these studies; however, the reduction in the risk of developing obesity observed in the two largest studies was substantial (20–37%). Promoting breastfeeding has many benefits, the prevention of childhood obesity probably being one of them.

Possible etiological factors
Several other factors were defined as "possible" protective or causative in the etiology of unhealthy weight gain.

Low-glycaemic foods have been proposed as a potential protective factor against weight gain and there are some early studies that support this hypothesis. More clinical trials are, however, needed to establish the association with greater certainty.

Large portion sizes are a possible causative factor for unhealthy weight gain (24). The marketing of "supersize" portions, particularly in fast-food outlets, is now common practice in many countries. There is some evidence that people poorly estimate portion sizes and that subsequent energy compensation for a large meal is incomplete and therefore is likely to lead to overconsumption.

In many countries, there has been a steady increase in the proportion of food eaten that is prepared outside the home. In the United States, the energy, total fat, saturated fat, cholesterol and sodium content of foods prepared outside the home is significantly higher than that of home-prepared food. People in the United States who tend to eat in restaurants have a higher BMI than those who tend to eat at home (25).

Certain psychological parameters of eating patterns may influence the risk of obesity. The "flexible restraint" pattern is associated with lower risk of weight gain, whereas the "rigid restraint/periodic disinhibition" pattern is associated with a higher risk.

Several other factors were also considered but the evidence was not thought to be strong enough to warrant defining them as protective or causative. Studies have not shown consistent associations between alcohol intake and obesity despite the high energy density of the nutrient (7 kcal/g). There are probably many confounding factors that influence the association. While a high eating frequency has been shown in some studies to have a negative relationship with energy intake and weight gain, the types of foods readily available as snack foods are often high in fat and a high consumption of foods of this type might predispose people to weight gain. The evidence regarding the impact of early nutrition on subsequent obesity is also mixed, with some studies showing relationships for high and low birth weights.

5.2.5 General strategies for obesity prevention

The prevention of obesity in infants and young children should be considered of high priority. For infants and young children, the main preventive strategies are:

— the promotion of exclusive breastfeeding;

— avoiding the use of added sugars and starches when feeding formula;

— instructing mothers to accept their child's ability to regulate energy intake rather than feeding until the plate is empty;

— assuring the appropriate micronutrient intake needed to promote optimal linear growth.

For children and adolescents, prevention of obesity implies the need to:

— promote an active lifestyle;

— limit television viewing;

— promote the intake of fruits and vegetables;

— restrict the intake of energy-dense, micronutrient-poor foods (e.g. packaged snacks);

— restrict the intake of sugars-sweetened soft drinks.

Additional measures include modifying the environment to enhance physical activity in schools and communities, creating more opportunities for family interaction (e.g. eating family meals), limiting the exposure of young children to heavy marketing practices of energy-dense, micronutrient-poor foods, and providing the necessary information and skills to make healthy food choices.

In developing countries, special attention should be given to avoidance of overfeeding stunted population groups. Nutrition programmes designed to control or prevent undernutrition need to assess stature in combination with weight to prevent providing excess energy to children of low weight-for-age but normal weight-for-height. In countries in economic transition, as populations become more sedentary and able to access energy-dense foods, there is a need to maintain the healthy components of traditional diets (e.g. high intake of vegetables, fruits and NSP). Education provided to mothers and low socioeconomic status communities that are food insecure should stress that overweight and obesity do not represent good health.

Low-income groups globally and populations in countries in economic transition often replace traditional micronutrient-rich foods by heavily marketed, sugars-sweetened beverages (i.e. soft drinks) and energy-dense fatty, salty and sugary foods. These trends, coupled with reduced physical activity, are associated with the rising prevalence of obesity. Strategies are needed to improve the quality of diets by increasing consumption of fruits and vegetables, in addition to increasing physical activity, in order to stem the epidemic of obesity and associated diseases.

5.2.6 *Disease-specific recommendations*

Body mass index (BMI)
BMI can be used to estimate, albeit crudely, the prevalence of overweight and obesity within a population and the risks associated with it. It does not, however, account for the wide variations in obesity between different individuals and populations. The classification of overweight and obesity, according to BMI, is shown in Table 8.

Table 8
Classification of overweight in adults according to BMI[a]

Classification	BMI (kg/m^2)	Risk of comorbidities
Underweight	<18.5	Low (but risk of other clinical problems increased)
Normal range	18.5–24.9	Average
Overweight	$\geqslant$25.0	
Pre-obese	25.0–29.9	Increased
Obese class I	30.0–34.9	Moderate
Obese class II	35.0–39.9	Severe
Obese class III	$\geqslant$40.0	Very severe

[a] These BMI values are age-independent and the same for both sexes. However, BMI may not correspond to the same degree of fatness in different populations due, in part, to differences in body proportions. The table shows a simplistic relationship between BMI and the risk of comorbidity, which can be affected by a range of factors, including the nature and the risk of comorbidity, which can be affected by a range of factors, including the nature of the diet, ethnic group and activity level. The risks associated with increasing BMI are continuous and graded and begin at a BMI below 25. The interpretation of BMI gradings in relation to risk may differ for different populations. Both BMI and a measure of fat distribution (waist circumference or waist : hip ratio (WHR)) are important in calculating the risk of obesity comorbidities.
Source: reference 26.

In recent years, different ranges of BMI cut-off points for overweight and obesity have been proposed, in particular for the Asia-Pacific region (27). At present available data on which to base definitive recommendations are sparse.[1] Nevertheless, the consultation considered that, to achieve optimum health, the median BMI for the adult population should be in the range 21–23 kg/m^2, while the goal for individuals should be to maintain BMI in the range 18.5–24.9 kg/m^2.

Waist circumference

Waist circumference is a convenient and simple measure which is unrelated to height, correlates closely with BMI and the ratio of waist-to-hip circumference, and is an approximate index of intra-abdominal fat mass and total body fat. Furthermore, changes in waist circumference reflect changes in risk factors for cardiovascular disease and other forms of chronic diseases, even though the risks seem to vary in different populations. There is an increased risk of metabolic complications for men with a waist circumference $\geqslant$102 cm, and women with a waist circumference $\geqslant$88 cm.

[1] A WHO Expert Consultation on Appropriate BMI for Asian Populations and its Implications for Policy and Intervention Strategies was held in Singapore from 8 to 11 July 2002 in order to: (i) review the scientific evidence on the relationship between BMI, body composition and risk factors in Asian populations; (ii) examine if population specific BMI cut-off points for overweight and obesity are necessary for Asian populations; (iii) examine the purpose and basis of ethnic-specific definitions; and iv) examine further research needs in this area. As one of its recommendations, the Consultation formed a Working Group to examine available data on the relationship between waist circumference and morbidity, and the interaction between BMI, waist circumference and health risk in order to define future research needs and develop recommendations for the use of additional waist measurements to further define risks.

Physical activity

A total of one hour per day of moderate-intensity activity, such as walking on most days of the week, is probably needed to maintain a healthy body weight, particularly for people with sedentary occupations.[2]

Total energy intake

The fat and water content of foods are the main determinants of the energy density of the diet. A lower consumption of energy-dense (i.e. high-fat, high-sugars and high-starch) foods and energy-dense (i.e. high free sugars) drinks contributes to a reduction in total energy intake. Conversely, a higher intake of energy-dilute foods (i.e. vegetables and fruits) and foods high in NSP (i.e. wholegrain cereals) contributes to a reduction in total energy intake and an improvement in micronutrient intake. It should be noted, however, that very active groups who have diets high in vegetables, legumes, fruits and wholegrain cereals, may sustain a total fat intake of up to 35% without the risk of unhealthy weight gain.

References

1. Colditz G. Economic costs of obesity and inactivity. *Medicine and Science in Sport and Exercise*, 1999, **31**(Suppl. 11):S663–S667.

2. *The world health report 2002: reducing risks, promoting healthy life*. Geneva, World Health Organization, 2002.

3. Manson JE et al. Body weight and mortality among women. *New England Journal of Medicine*, 1995, **333**:677–685.

4. Fogelholm M, Kukkonen-Harjula K. Does physical activity prevent weight gain – a systematic review. *Obesity Reviews*, 2000, **1**:95–111.

5. *Weight control and physical activity*. Lyon, International Agency for Research on Cancer, 2002 (IARC Handbooks of Cancer Prevention, Vol. 6).

6. Saris WHM. Dose–response of physical activity in the treatment of obesity–How much is enough to prevent unhealthy weight gain. Outcome of the First Mike Stock Conference. *International Journal of Obesity*, 2002, **26**(Suppl. 1):S108.

7. Pereira MA, Ludwig DS. Dietary fiber and body-weight regulation. Observations and mechanisms. *Pediatric Clinics of North America*, 2001, **48**:969–980.

8. Howarth NC, Saltzman E, Roberts SB. Dietary fiber and weight regulation. *Nutrition Reviews*, 2001, **59**:129–139.

9. Astrup A et al. The role of low-fat diets in body weight control: a meta-analysis of ad libitum dietary intervention studies. *International Journal of Obesity*, 2000, **24**:1545–1552.

10. Willett WC. Dietary fat plays a major role in obesity: no. *Obesity Reviews*, 2000, **3**:59–68.

---

[2] See also reference 5.

11. Campbell K, Crawford D. Family food environments as determinants of preschool-aged children's eating behaviours: implications for obesity prevention policy. A review. *Australian Journal of Nutrition and Dietetics*, 2001, **58**:19–25.

12. Gortmaker S et al. Reducing obesity via a school-based interdisciplinary intervention among youth: Planet Health. *Archives of Pediatrics and Adolescent Medicine*, 1999, **153**:409–418.

13. Nestle M. *Food politics.* Berkeley, CA, University of California Press, 2002.

14. Nestle M. The ironic politics of obesity. *Science, 2003,* **299**:781.

15. Robinson TN. Does television cause childhood obesity? *Journal of American Medical Association*, 1998, **279**:959–960.

16. Borzekowski DL, Robinson TN. The 30-second effect: an experiment revealing the impact of television commercials on food preferences of preschoolers. *Journal of the American Dietetic Association, 2001,* **101**:42–46.

17. Lewis MK, Hill AJ. Food advertising on British children's television: a content analysis and experimental study with nine-year olds. *International Journal of Obesity*, 1998, **22**:206–214.

18. Taras HL, Gage M. Advertised foods on children's television. *Archives of Pediatrics and Adolescent Medicine*, 1995, **149**:649–652.

19. Mattes RD. Dietary compensation by humans for supplemental energy provided as ethanol or carbohydrate in fluids. *Physiology and Behaviour*, 1996, **59**:179–187.

20. Tordoff MG, Alleva AM. Effect of drinking soda sweetened with aspartame or high-fructose corn syrup on food intake and body weight. *American Journal of Clinical Nutrition*, 1990, **51**:963–969.

21. Harnack L, Stang J, Story M. Soft drink consumption among US children and adolescents: nutritional consequences. *Journal of the American Dietetic Association*, 1999, **99**:436–441.

22. Ludwig DS, Peterson KE, Gortmaker SL. Relation between consumption of sugar-sweetened drinks and childhood obesity: a prospective, observational analysis. *Lancet*, 2001, **357**:505–508.

23. Peña M, Bacallao J. *Obesity and poverty: a new public health challenge.* Washington, DC, Pan American Health Organization, 2000 (Scientific Publication, No. 576).

24. Nielsen SJ, Popkin BM. Patterns and trends in food portion sizes, 1977–1998. *Journal of the American Medical Association, 2003,* **289**:450–453.

25. Jeffery RW, French SA. Epidemic obesity in the United States: are fast foods and television viewing contributing? *American Journal of Public Health,* 1998, **88**:277–280.

26. *Obesity: preventing and managing the global epidemic. Report of a WHO Consultation.* Geneva, World Health Organization, 2000 (WHO Technical Report Series, No. 894).

27. WHO Regional Office for the Western Pacific/International Association for the Study of Obesity/International Obesity Task Force. *The Asia-Pacific perspective: redefining obesity and its treatment.* Sydney, Health Communications Australia, 2000.

5.3 Recommendations for preventing diabetes

5.3.1 *Background*

Type 2 diabetes, formerly known as non-insulin-dependent diabetes (NIDDM), accounts for most cases of diabetes worldwide. Type 2 diabetes develops when the production of insulin is insufficient to overcome the underlying abnormality of increased resistance to its action. The early stages of type 2 diabetes are characterized by overproduction of insulin. As the disease progresses, process insulin levels may fall as a result of partial failure of the insulin producing β cells of the pancreas. Complications of type 2 diabetes include blindness, kidney failure, foot ulceration which may lead to gangrene and subsequent amputation, and appreciably increased risk of infections, coronary heart disease and stroke. The enormous and escalating economic and social costs of type 2 diabetes make a compelling case for attempts to reduce the risk of developing the condition as well as for energetic management of the established disease (*1, 2*).

Lifestyle modification is the cornerstone of both treatment and attempts to prevent type 2 diabetes (*3*). The changes required to reduce the risk of developing type 2 diabetes at the population level are, however, unlikely to be achieved without major environmental changes to facilitate appropriate choices by individuals. Criteria for the diagnosis of type 2 diabetes and for the earlier stages in the disease process − impaired glucose tolerance and impaired fasting glucose − have recently been revised (*4, 5*).

Type 1 diabetes, previously known as insulin-dependent diabetes, occurs much less frequently and is associated with an absolute deficiency of insulin, usually resulting from autoimmune destruction of the β cells of the pancreas. Environmental as well as genetic factors appear to be involved but there is no convincing evidence of a role for lifestyle factors which can be modified to reduce the risk.

5.3.2 *Trends*

Although increases in both the prevalence and incidence of type 2 diabetes have occurred globally, they have been especially dramatic in societies in economic transition in much of the newly industrialized world and in developing countries (*1, 6–9*). Worldwide, the number of cases of diabetes is currently estimated to be around 150 million. This number is predicted to double by 2025, with the greatest number of cases being expected in China and India. These numbers may represent an underestimate and there are likely to be many undiagnosed cases. Previously a disease of the middle-aged and elderly, type 2 diabetes has recently escalated in all age groups and is now being identified in younger and younger age groups, including adolescents and children, especially in high-risk populations.

Age-adjusted mortality rates among people with diabetes are 1.5–2.5 times higher than in the general population (*10*). In Caucasian populations, much of the excess mortality is attributable to cardiovascular disease, especially coronary heart disease (*11, 12*); amongst Asian and American Indian populations, renal disease is a major contributor (*13, 14*), whereas in some developing nations, infections are an important cause of death (*15*). It is conceivable that the decline in mortality due to coronary heart disease which has occurred in many affluent societies may be halted or even reversed if rates of type 2 diabetes continue to increase. This may occur if the coronary risk factors associated with diabetes increase to the extent that the risk they mediate outweighs the benefit accrued from improvements in conventional cardiovascular risk factors and the improved care of patients with established cardiovascular disease (*3*).

5.3.3 *Diet, physical activity and diabetes*

Type 2 diabetes results from an interaction between genetic and environmental factors. The rapidly changing incidence rates, however, suggest a particularly important role for the latter as well as a potential for stemming the tide of the global epidemic of the disease. The most dramatic increases in type 2 diabetes are occurring in societies in which there have been major changes in the type of diet consumed, reductions in physical activity, and increases in overweight and obesity. The diets concerned are typically energy-dense, high in saturated fatty acids and depleted in NSP.

In all societies, overweight and obesity are associated with an increased risk of type 2 diabetes, especially when the excess adiposity is centrally distributed. Conventional (BMI) categories may not be an appropriate means of determining the risk of developing type 2 diabetes in individuals of all population groups because of ethnic differences in body composition and because of the importance of the distribution of excess adiposity. While all lifestyle-related and environmental factors which contribute to excess weight gain may be regarded as contributing to type 2 diabetes, the evidence that individual dietary factors have an effect which is independent of their obesity promoting effect, is inconclusive. Evidence that saturated fatty acids increase risk of type 2 diabetes and that NSP are protective is more convincing than the evidence for several other nutrients which have been implicated. The presence of maternal diabetes, including gestational diabetes and intrauterine growth retardation, especially when associated with later rapid catch-up growth, appears to increase the risk of subsequently developing diabetes.

5.3.4 *Strength of evidence*

The association between excessive weight gain, central adiposity and the development of type 2 diabetes is convincing. The association has been repeatedly demonstrated in longitudinal studies in different populations, with a striking gradient of risk apparent with increasing levels of BMI, adult weight gain, waist circumference or waist-to-hip ratio. Indeed waist circumference or waist-to-hip ratio (reflecting abdominal or visceral adiposity) are more powerful determinants of subsequent risk of type 2 diabetes than BMI (16–20). Central adiposity is also an important determinant of insulin resistance, the underlying abnormality in most cases of type 2 diabetes (20). Voluntary weight loss improves insulin sensitivity (21) and in several randomized controlled trials has been shown to reduce the risk of progression from impaired glucose tolerance to type 2 diabetes (22, 23).

Longitudinal studies have clearly indicated that increased physical activity reduces the risk of developing type 2 diabetes regardless of the degree of adiposity (24–26). Vigorous exercise (i.e. training to an intensity of 80–90% of age-predicted maximum heart rate for at least 20 minutes, at least five times per week) has the potential to substantially enhance insulin sensitivity (21). The minimum intensity and duration of physical activity required to improve insulin sensitivity has not been established.

Offspring of diabetic pregnancies (including gestational diabetes) are often large and heavy at birth, tend to develop obesity in childhood and are at high risk of developing type 2 diabetes at an early age (27). Those born to mothers after they have developed diabetes have a three-fold higher risk of developing diabetes than those born before (28).

In observational epidemiological studies, a high saturated fat intake has been associated with a higher risk of impaired glucose tolerance, and higher fasting glucose and insulin levels (29–32). Higher proportions of saturated fatty acids in serum lipid or muscle phospholipid have been associated with higher fasting insulin, lower insulin sensitivity and a higher risk of type 2 diabetes (33–35). Higher unsaturated fatty acids from vegetable sources and polyunsaturated fatty acids have been associated with a reduced risk of type 2 diabetes (36, 37) and lower fasting and 2-hour glucose concentrations (32, 38). Furthermore, higher proportions of long-chain polyunsaturated fatty acids in skeletal muscle phospholipids have been associated with increased insulin sensitivity (39).

In human intervention studies, replacement of saturated by unsaturated fatty acids leads to improved glucose tolerance (40, 41) and enhanced insulin sensitivity (42). Long-chain polyunsaturated fatty acids do not, however, appear to confer additional benefit over monounsaturated fatty acids in intervention studies (42). Furthermore, when total fat intake is high (greater than 37% of total energy), altering the quality of dietary fat appears to have little effect (42), a finding which is not surprising given that in observational studies a high intake of total fat has been shown to predict development of impaired glucose tolerance and the progression of impaired glucose tolerance to type 2 diabetes (29, 43). A high total fat intake has also been associated with higher fasting insulin concentrations and a lower insulin sensitivity index (44, 45).

Considered in aggregate these findings are deemed to indicate a probable causal link between saturated fatty acids and type 2 diabetes, and a possible causal association between total fat intake and type 2 diabetes. The two randomized controlled trials which showed a potential for lifestyle modification to reduce the risk of progression from impaired glucose tolerance to type 2 diabetes included advice to reduce total and saturated fat (22, 23), but in both trials it is impossible to disentangle the effects of individual dietary manipulation.

Research relating to the association between NSP intake and type 2 diabetes is complicated by ambiguity with regard to the definitions used (the term dietary fibre and NSP are often incorrectly used interchangeably), different methods of analysis and, consequently, inconsistencies in food composition tables. Observations by Trowell in Uganda more than 30 years ago suggested that the infrequency of diabetes in rural Africa may be the result of a protective effect of substantial amounts of NSP in the diet (referred to as dietary fibre) associated with a high consumption of minimally-processed or unprocessed carbohydrate. The author also hypothesized that through-out the world, increasing intakes of highly-processed carbohydrate, depleted in NSP, had promoted the development of diabetes (46). Three cohort studies (the Health Professionals Follow-up Study of men aged 40–75 years, the Nurses' Health Study of women aged 40–65 years, and the Iowa Women's Health Study in women aged 55–69 years) have shown a protective effect of NSP (dietary fibre) (47–49) which was independent of age, BMI, smoking and physical activity. In many controlled experimental studies, high intakes of NSP (dietary fibre) have repeatedly been shown to result in reduced blood glucose and insulin levels in people with type 2 diabetes and impaired glucose tolerance (50). Moreover an increased intake of wholegrain cereals, vegetables and fruits (all rich in NSP) was a feature of the diets associated with a reduced risk of progression of impaired glucose tolerance to type 2 diabetes in the two randomized controlled trials previously described (22, 23). Thus the evidence for a potential protective effect of NSP (dietary fibre) appears strong. However, the fact that the experimental studies suggest that soluble forms of NSP exert benefit (50–53) whereas the prospective cohort studies suggest that it is the cereal-derived insoluble forms that are protective (47, 48) explain the "probable" rather "convincing" grading of the level of evidence.

Many foods which are rich in NSP (especially soluble forms), such as pulses, have a low glycaemic index.[1] Other carbohydrate-containing foods (e.g. certain types of pasta), which are not especially high in NSP, also have a low glycaemic index. Low glycaemic index foods, regardless of their NSP content, are not only associated with a reduced glycaemic response after ingestion when compared with foods of higher glycaemic index, but are also associated with an overall improvement in glycaemic control (as measured by haemoglobin A_1c) in people with diabetes (54–57). A low glycaemic index does not, however, per se, confer overall health benefits, since a high fat or fructose content of a food may also result in a reduced glycaemic index and such foods may also be energy-dense. Thus while this property of carbohydrate-containing foods may well influence the risk of developing type 2 diabetes, the evidence is accorded a lower level of strength than the evidence relating to the NSP content. Similarly, the level of evidence for the protective effect of n-3 fatty acids is regarded as "possible" because the results of epidemiological studies are inconsistent and the experimental data inconclusive. There is insufficient evidence to confirm or refute the suggestions that chromium, magnesium, vitamin E and moderate intakes of alcohol might protect against the development of type 2 diabetes.

A number of studies, mostly in developing countries, have suggested that intrauterine growth retardation and low birth weight are associated with subsequent development of insulin resistance (58). In those countries where there has been chronic undernutrition, insulin resistance may have been selectively advantageous in terms of surviving famine. In populations where energy intake has increased and lifestyles have become more sedentary, however, insulin resistance and the consequent risk of type 2 diabetes have been enhanced. In particular, rapid postnatal catch-up growth appears to further increase the risk of type 2 diabetes in later life. Appropriate strategies which may help to reduce type 2 diabetes risk in this situation include improving the nutrition of young children, promoting linear growth and preventing energy excess by limiting intake of energy-dense foods, controlling the quality of fat supply, and facilitating physical activity. At a population level, fetal growth may remain restricted until maternal height improves. This may take several generations to correct. The prevention of type 2 diabetes in infants and young children may be facilitated by the promotion of exclusive breastfeeding, avoiding overweight and obesity, and promoting optimum linear growth. The strength of evidence on lifestyle factors is summarized in Table 9.

---

[1] The glycaemic index is calculated as the glycaemic response to a quantity of food containing a set amount, usually 50 g, of carbohydrate, expressed as a percentage of the glycaemic response following ingestion of a similar quantity of glucose or of carbohydrate in white bread.

Table 9
Summary of strength of evidence on lifestyle factors and risk of developing type 2 diabetes

Evidence	Decreased risk	No relationship	Increased risk
Convincing	Voluntary weight loss in overweight and obese people Physical activity		Overweight and obesity Abdominal obesity Physical inactivity Maternal diabetes[a]
Probable	NSP		Saturated fats Intrauterine growth retardation
Possible	n-3 fatty acids Low glycaemic index foods Exclusive breastfeeding[b]		Total fat intake Trans fatty acids
Insufficient	Vitamin E Chromium Magnesium Moderate alcohol		Excess alcohol

[1] NSP, non-starch polysaccharides.
[a] Includes gestational diabetes.
[b] As a global public health recommendation, infants should be exclusively breastfed for the first six months of life to achieve optimal growth, development and health (59).

5.3.5 *Disease-specific recommendations*

Measures aimed at reducing overweight and obesity, and cardiovascular disease are likely to also reduce the risk of developing type 2 diabetes and its complications. Some measures are particularly relevant to reducing the risk for diabetes; these are listed below:

- Prevention/treatment of overweight and obesity, particularly in high-risk groups.
- Maintaining an optimum BMI, i.e. at the lower end of the normal range. For the adult population, this means maintaining a mean BMI in the range 21–23 kg/m^2 and avoiding weight gain (> 5 kg) in adult life.
- Voluntary weight reduction in overweight or obese individuals with impaired glucose tolerance (although screening for such individuals may not be cost-effective in many countries).
- Practising an endurance activity at moderate or greater level of intensity (e.g. brisk walking) for one hour or more per day on most days per week.
- Ensuring that saturated fat intake does not exceed 10% of total energy and for high-risk groups, fat intake should be $< 7\%$ of total energy.
- Achieving adequate intakes of NSP through regular consumption of wholegrain cereals, legumes, fruits and vegetables. A minimum daily intake of 20 g is recommended.

References

1. King H, Aubert RE, Herman WH. Global burden of diabetes, 1995–2025: prevalence, numerical estimates, and projections. *Diabetes Care*, 1998, **21**:1414–1431.

2. Amos AF, McCarty DJ, Zimmet P. The rising global burden of diabetes and its complications: estimates and projections to the year 2010. *Diabetic Medicine*, 1997, **14**(Suppl. 5):S1–S85.

3. Mann J. Stemming the tide of diabetes mellitus. *Lancet*, 2000, **356**:1454–1455.

4. Report of the Expert Committee on the Diagnosis and Classification of Diabetes Mellitus. *Diabetes Care*, 1997, **20**:1183–1197.

5. *Definition, diagnosis and classification of diabetes mellitus and its complications. Report of a WHO Consultation. Part 1. Diagnosis and classification of diabetes mellitus.* Geneva, World Health Organization, 1999 (document WHO/NCD/NCS/99.2).

6. Harris MI et al. Prevalence of diabetes, impaired fasting glucose, and impaired glucose tolerance in U.S. adults. The Third National Health and Nutrition Examination Survey, 1988–1994. *Diabetes Care*, 1998, **21**:518–524.

7. Flegal KM et al. Prevalence of diabetes in Mexican Americans, Cubans, and Puerto Ricans from the Hispanic Health and Nutrition Examination Survey, 1982–1984. *Diabetes Care*, 1991, **14**:628–638.

8. Mokdad AH et al. Diabetes trends among American Indians and Alaska natives: 1990–1998. *Diabetes Care*, 2001, **24**:1508–1509.

9. Mokdad AH et al. The continuing epidemics of obesity and diabetes in the United States. *Journal of the American Medical Association*, 2001, **286**:1195–1200.

10. Kleinman JC et al. Mortality among diabetics in a national sample. *American Journal of Epidemiology*, 1988, **128**:389–401.

11. Gu K, Cowie CC, Harris MI. Mortality in adults with and without diabetes in a national cohort of the US population, 1971–1993. *Diabetes Care*, 1998, **21**:1138–1145.

12. Roper NA et al. Excess mortality in a population with diabetes and the impact of material deprivation: longitudinal, population-based study. *British Medical Journal*, 2001, **322**:1389–1393.

13. Morrish et al. Mortality and causes of death in the WHO Multinational Study of Vascular Disease in Diabetes. *Diabetologia*, 2001, **44**(Suppl. 2):S14–S21.

14. Sievers ML et al. Impact of NIDDM on mortality and causes of death in Pima Indians. *Diabetes Care*, 1992, **15**:1541–1549.

15. McLarty DG, Kinabo L, Swai AB. Diabetes in tropical Africa: a prospective study, 1981–7. II. Course and prognosis. *British Medical Journal*, 1990, **300**:1107–1110.

16. Colditz GA et al. Weight as a risk factor for clinical diabetes in women. *American Journal of Epidemiology*, 1990, **132**:501–513.

17. Després JP et al. Treatment of obesity: need to focus on high-risk abdominally obese patients. *British Medical Journal*, 2001, **322**:716-720.

18. Chan JM et al. Obesity, fat distribution, and weight gain as risk factors for clinical diabetes in men. *Diabetes Care*, 1994, **17**:961–969.

19. Boyko EJ et al. Visceral adiposity and risk of type 2 diabetes: a prospective study among Japanese Americans. *Diabetes Care*, 2000, **23**:465–471.

20. Després JP. Health consequences of visceral obesity. *Annals of Medicine*, 2001, **33**:534–541.

21. McAuley KA et al. Intensive lifestyle changes are necessary to improve insulin sensitivity. *Diabetes Care*, 2002, **25**:445–452.

22. Tuomilehto J et al. Prevention of type 2 diabetes mellitus by changes in lifestyle among subjects with impaired glucose tolerance. *New England Journal of Medicine*, 2002, **344**:1343–1350.

23. Knowler WC et al. Reduction in the incidence of type 2 diabetes with lifestyle intervention of metformin. *New England Journal of Medicine*, 2002, **346**:393–403.

24. Manson JE et al. A prospective study of exercise and incidence of diabetes among US male physicians. *Journal of the American Medical Association*, 1992, **268**:63–67.

25. Kriska AM et al. The association of physical activity with obesity, fat distribution and glucose intolerance in Pima Indians. *Diabetologia*, 1993, **36**:863–869.

26. Helmrich SP et al. Physical activity and reduced occurrence of non-insulin-dependent diabetes mellitus. *New England Journal of Medicine*, 1991, **325**:147–152.

27. Pettitt DJ et al. Congenital susceptibility to NIDDM. Role of intrauterine environment. *Diabetes*, 1988, **37**:622–628.

28. Dabelea D et al. Intrauterine exposure to diabetes conveys risks for type 2 diabetes and obesity: a study of discordant sibships. *Diabetes*, 2000, **49**:2208–2211.

29. Feskens EJM et al. Dietary factors determining diabetes and impaired glucose tolerance. A 20-year follow-up of the Finnish and Dutch cohorts of the Seven Countries Study. *Diabetes Care*, 1995, **18**:1104–1112.

30. Bo S et al. Dietary fat and gestational hyperglycaemia. *Diabetologia*, 2001, **44**:972–978.

31. Feskens EJM, Kromhout D. Habitual dietary intake and glucose tolerance in euglycaemic men: the Zutphen Study. *International Journal of Epidemiology*, 1990, **19**:953–959.

32. Parker DR et al. Relationship of dietary saturated fatty acids and body habitus to serum insulin concentrations: the Normative Aging Study. *American Journal of Clinical Nutrition*, 1993, **58**:129–136.

33. Folsom AR et al. Relation between plasma phospholipid saturated fatty acids and hyperinsulinemia. *Metabolism*, 1996, **45**:223–228.

34. Vessby B, Tengblad S, Lithell H. Insulin sensitivity is related to the fatty acid composition of serum lipids and skeletal muscle phospholipids in 70-year-old men. *Diabetologia*, 1994, **37**:1044–1050.

35. Vessby B et al. The risk to develop NIDDM is related to the fatty acid composition of the serum cholesterol esters. *Diabetes*, 1994, **43**:1353–1357.

36. Salmeron J et al. Dietary fat intake and risk of type 2 diabetes in women. *American Journal of Clinical Nutrition*, 2001, **73**:1019–1026.

37. Meyer KA et al. Dietary fat and incidence of type 2 diabetes in older Iowa women. *Diabetes Care*, 2001, **24**:1528–1535.

38. Mooy JM et al. Prevalence and determinants of glucose intolerance in a Dutch Caucasian population. The Hoorn Study. *Diabetes Care*, 1995, **18**:1270–1273.

39. Pan DA et al. Skeletal muscle membrane lipid composition is related to adiposity and insulin action. *Journal of Clinical Investigation*, 1995, **96**:2802–2808.

40. Uusitupa M et al. Effects of two high-fat diets with different fatty acid compositions on glucose and lipid metabolism in healthy young women. *American Journal of Clinical Nutrition,* 1994, **59**:1310–1316.

41. Vessby B et al. Substituting polyunsaturated for saturated fat as a single change in a Swedish diet: effects on serum lipoprotein metabolism and glucose tolerance in patients with hyperlipoproteinaemia. *European Journal of Clinical Investigation,* 1980, **10**:193–202.

42. Vessby B et al. Substituting dietary saturated for monounsaturated fat impairs insulin sensitivity in healthy men and women: the KANWU Study. *Diabetologia,* 2001, **44**:312–319.

43. Marshall JA et al. Dietary fat predicts conversion from impaired glucose tolerance to NIDDM. The San Luis Valley Diabetes Study. *Diabetes Care,* 1994, **17**:50–56.

44. Mayer EJ et al. Usual dietary fat intake and insulin concentrations in healthy women twins. *Diabetes Care,* 1993, **16**:1459–1469.

45. Lovejoy J, DiGirolamo M. Habitual dietary intake and insulin sensitivity in lean and obese adults. *American Journal of Clinical Nutrition,* 1992, **55**:1174–1179.

46. Trowell HC. Dietary-fiber hypothesis of the etiology of diabetes mellitus. *Diabetes,* 1975, **24**:762–765.

47. Salmeron J et al. Dietary fiber, glycemic load and risk of NIDDM in men. *Diabetes Care,* 1997, **20**:545–550.

48. Salmeron J et al. Dietary fiber, glycemic load, and risk of non-insulin-dependent diabetes mellitus in women. *Journal of the American Medical Association,* 1997, **277**:472–477.

49. Meyer KA et al. Carbohydrates, dietary fiber, and incident type 2 diabetes in older women. *American Journal of Clinical Nutrition,* 2000, **71**:921–930.

50. Mann J. Dietary fibre and diabetes revisited. *European Journal of Clinical Nutrition,* 2001, **55**:919–921.

51. Simpson HRC et al. A high carbohydrate leguminous fibre diet improves all aspects of diabetic control. *Lancet,* 1981, **1**:1–5.

52. Mann J. Lawrence lecture. Lines to legumes: changing concepts of diabetic diets. *Diabetic Medicine,* 1984, **1**:191–198.

53. Chandalia M et al. Beneficial effects of high dietary fiber intake in patients with type 2 diabetes mellitus. *New England Journal of Medicine,* 2000, **342**:1392–1398.

54. Frost G, Wilding J, Beecham J. Dietary advice based on the glycaemic index improves dietary profile and metabolic control in type 2 diabetic patients. *Diabetic Medicine,* 1994, **11**:397–401.

55. Brand JC et al. Low-glycemic index foods improve long-term glycemic control in NIDDM. *Diabetes Care,* 1991, **14**:95–101.

56. Fontvieille AM et al. The use of low glycaemic index foods improves metabolic control of diabetic patients over five weeks. *Diabetic Medicine,* 1992, **9**:444–450.

57. Wolever TMS et al. Beneficial effect of a low glycaemic index diet in type 2 diabetes. *Diabetic Medicine,* 1992, **9**:451–458.

58. Stern MP et al. Birth weight and the metabolic syndrome: thrifty phenotype or thrifty genotype? *Diabetes/Metabolism Research and Reviews,* 2000, **16**:88–93.

59. *Infant and young child nutrition.* Geneva, World Health Organization, 2001 (document A54/2).

5.4 Recommendations for preventing cardiovascular diseases

5.4.1 *Background*

The second half of the 20th century has witnessed major shifts in the pattern of disease, in addition to marked improvements in life expectancy, this period is characterized by profound changes in diet and lifestyles which in turn have contributed to an epidemic of noncommunicable diseases. This epidemic is now emerging, and even accelerating, in most developing countries, while infections and nutritional deficiencies are receding as leading contributors to death and disability (*1*).

In developing countries, the effect of the nutrition transition and the concomitant rise in the prevalence of cardiovascular diseases will be to widen the mismatch between health care needs and resources, and already scarce resources will be stretched ever more thinly. Because unbalanced diets, obesity and physical inactivity all contribute to heart disease, addressing these, along with tobacco use, can help to stem the epidemic. A large measure of success in this area has already been demonstrated in many industrialized countries.

5.4.2 *Trends*

Cardiovascular diseases are the major contributor to the global burden of disease among the noncommunicable diseases. WHO currently attributes one-third of all global deaths (15.3 million) to CVD, with developing countries, low-income and middle-income countries accounting for 86% of the DALYs lost to CVD worldwide in 1998. In the next two decades the increasing burden of CVD will be borne mostly by developing countries.

5.4.3 *Diet, physical activity and cardiovascular disease*

The "lag-time" effect of risk factors for CVD means that present mortality rates are the consequence of previous exposure to behavioural risk factors such as inappropriate nutrition, insufficient physical activity and increased tobacco consumption. Overweight, central obesity, high blood pressure, dyslipidaemia, diabetes and low cardio-respiratory fitness are among the biological factors contributing principally to increased risk. Unhealthy dietary practices include the high consumption of saturated fats, salt and refined carbohydrates, as well as low consumption of fruits and vegetables, and these tend to cluster together.

5.4.4 *Strength of evidence*

Convincing associations for reduced risk of CVD include consumption of fruits (including berries) and vegetables, fish and fish oils (eicosapentaenoic acid (EPA) and docosahexaenoic acid (DHA)), foods high in linoleic acid and potassium, as well as physical activity and low to moderate alcohol intake. While vitamin E intake appears to have no relationship to risk of CVD, there is convincing evidence that myristic and palmitic acids, trans fatty acids, high sodium intake, overweight and high alcohol intake contribute to an increase in risk. A "probable" level of evidence demonstrates a decreased risk for α-linolenic acid, oleic acid, NSP, wholegrain cereals, nuts (unsalted), folate, plant sterols and stanols, and no relationship for stearic acid. There is a probable increase in risk from dietary cholesterol and unfiltered boiled coffee. Possible associations for reduced risk include intake of flavonoids and consumption of soy products, while possible associations for increased risk include fats rich in lauric acid, β-carotene supplements and impaired fetal nutrition. The evidence supporting these conclusions is summarized below.

Fatty acids and dietary cholesterol
The relationship between dietary fats and CVD, especially coronary heart disease, has been extensively investigated, with strong and consistent associations emerging from a wide body of evidence accrued from animal experiments, as well as observational studies, clinical trials and metabolic studies conducted in diverse human populations (*2*).

Saturated fatty acids raise total and low-density lipoprotein (LDL) cholesterol, but individual fatty acids within this group, have different effects (*3–5*). Myristic and palmitic acids have the greatest effect and are abundant in diets rich in dairy products and meat. Stearic acid has not been shown to elevate blood cholesterol and is rapidly converted to oleic acid in vivo. The most effective replacement for saturated fatty acids in terms of coronary heart disease outcome are polyunsaturated fatty acids, especially linoleic acid. This finding is supported by the results of several large randomized clinical trials, in which replacement of saturated and trans fatty acids by polyunsaturated vegetable oils lowered coronary heart disease risk (*6*).

Trans fatty acids are geometrical isomers of cis-unsaturated fatty acids that adapt a saturated fatty acid-like configuration. Partial hydrogenation, the process used to increase shelf-life of polyunsaturated fatty acids (PUFAs) creates trans fatty acids and also removes the critical double bonds in essential fatty acids necessary for the action. Metabolic studies have demonstrated that trans fatty acids render the plasma lipid profile even more atherogenic than saturated fatty acids, by not only elevating LDL cholesterol to similar levels but also by decreasing high-density lipoprotein (HDL) cholesterol (*7*). Several large cohort studies have found that intake of trans fatty acids increases the risk of coronary heart disease (*8, 9*). Most trans fatty acids are contributed by industrially hardened oils. Even though trans fatty acids have been reduced or eliminated from retail fats and spreads in many parts of the world, deep-fried fast foods and baked goods are a major and increasing source (7).

When substituted for saturated fatty acids in metabolic studies, both monounsaturated fatty acids and n-6 polyunsaturated fatty acids lower plasma total and LDL cholesterol concentrations (10); PUFAs are somewhat more effective than monounsaturates in this respect. The only nutritionally important monounsaturated fatty acids is oleic acid, which is abundant in olive and canola oils and also in nuts. The most important polyunsaturated fatty acid is linoleic acid, which is abundant especially in soybean and sunflower oils. The most important n-3 PUFAs are eicosapentaenoic acid and docosahexaenoic acid found in fatty fish, and α-linolenic acid found in plant foods. The biological effects of n-3 PUFAs are wide ranging, involving lipids and lipoproteins, blood pressure, cardiac function, arterial compliance, endothelial function, vascular reactivity and cardiac electrophysiology, as well as potent anti-platelet and anti-inflammatory effects (11). The very long chain n-3 PUFAs (eicosapentaenoic acid and docosahexaenoic acid) powerfully lower serum triglycerides but they raise serum LDL cholesterol. Therefore, their effect on coronary heart disease is probably mediated through pathways other than serum cholesterol.

Most of the epidemiological evidence related to n-3 PUFAs is derived from studies of fish consumption in populations or interventions involving fish diets in clinical trials (evidence on fish consumption is discussed further below). Fish oils have been used in the Gruppo Italiano per lo Studio della Sopravvivenza nell'Infarto Miocardico (GISSI) trial involving survivors of myocardial infarction (12). After 3.5 years of follow-up, the group that received fish oil had a 20% reduction in total mortality, a 30% reduction in cardiovascular death and a 45% decrease in sudden death. Several prospective studies have found an inverse association between the intake of α-linolenic acid, (high in flaxseed, canola and soybean oils), and risk of fatal coronary heart disease (13, 14).

Cholesterol in the blood and tissues is derived from two sources: diet and endogenous synthesis. Dairy fat and meat are major dietary sources. Egg yolk is particularly rich in cholesterol but unlike dairy products and meat does not provide saturated fatty acids. Although dietary cholesterol raises plasma cholesterol levels (15), observational evidence for an association of dietary cholesterol intake with CVD is contradictory (16). There is no requirement for dietary cholesterol and it is advisable to keep the intake as low as possible (2). If intake of dairy fat and meat are controlled, there is no need to severely restrict egg yolk intake, although some limitation remains prudent.

Dietary plant sterols, especially sitostanol, reduce serum cholesterol by inhibiting cholesterol absorption (*17*). The cholesterol-lowering effects of plant sterols has also been well documented (*18*) and commercial products made of these compounds are widely available, but their long-term effects remain to be seen.

NSP (dietary fibre)

Dietary fibre is a heterogeneous mixture of polysaccharides and lignin that cannot be degraded by the endogenous enzymes of vertebrate animals. Water-soluble fibres include pectins, gums, mucilages and some hemicelluloses. Insoluble fibres include cellulose and other hemicelluloses. Most fibres reduce plasma total and LDL cholesterol, as reported by several trials (*19*). Several large cohort studies carried out in different countries have reported that a high fibre diet as well as a diet high in wholegrain cereals lowers the risk of coronary heart disease (*20–23*).

Antioxidants, folate, and flavonoids

Even though antioxidants could, in theory, be protective against CVD and there is observational data supporting this theory, controlled trials employing supplements have been disappointing. The Heart Outcomes Prevention Evaluation trial (HOPE), a definitive clinical trial relating vitamin E supplementation to CVD outcomes, revealed no effect of vitamin E supplementation on myocardial infarction, stroke or death from cardiovascular causes in men or women (*24*). Also, the results of the Heart Protection Study indicated that no significant benefits of daily supplementation of vitamin E, vitamin C and β-carotene were observed among the high-risk individuals that were the subject of the study (*25*). In several studies where dietary vitamin C reduced the risk of coronary heart disease, supplemental vitamin C had little effect. Clinical trial evidence is lacking at present. Observational cohort studies have suggested a protective role for carotenoids but a meta-analysis of four randomized trials, in contrast, reported an increased risk of cardiovascular death (*26*).

The relationship of folate to CVD has been mostly explored through its effect on homocysteine, which may itself be an independent risk factor for coronary heart disease and probably also for stroke. Folic acid is required for the methylation of homocysteine to methionine. Reduced plasma folate has been strongly associated with elevated plasma homocysteine levels and folate supplementation has been demonstrated to decrease those levels (*27*). However, the role of homocysteine as an independent risk factor for CVD has been subject to much debate, since several prospective studies have not found this association to be independent of other risk factors (*28, 29*). It has also been suggested that elevation of plasma homocysteine is a consequence and not a cause of atherosclerosis, wherein impaired renal function resulting from atherosclerosis raises plasma homocysteine levels (*30, 31*). Data from the Nurses' Health Study showed that folate and vitamin B6, from diet and supplements, conferred protection against coronary heart disease (*32*). A recently published meta-analysis concluded that a higher intake of folate (0.8 mg folic acid) would reduce the risk of ischaemic heart disease by 16% and stroke by 24% (*33*).

Flavonoids are polyphenolic compounds that occur in a variety of foods of vegetable origin, such as tea, onions and apples. Data from several prospective studies indicate an inverse association of dietary flavonoids with coronary heart disease (*34, 35*). However, confounding may be a major problem and may explain the conflicting results of observational studies.

Sodium and potassium
High blood pressure is a major risk factor for coronary heart disease and both forms of stroke (ischaemic and haemorrhagic). Of the many risk factors associated with high blood pressure, the dietary exposure that has been most investigated is daily sodium intake. It has been studied extensively in animal experimental models, in epidemiological studies, controlled clinical trials and in population studies on restricted sodium intake (*36, 37*).

All these data show convincingly that sodium intake is directly associated with blood pressure. An overview of observational data obtained from population studies suggested that a difference in sodium intake of 100 mmol per day was associated with average differences in systolic blood pressure of 5 mmHg at age 15–19 years and 10 mmHg at age 60–69 years (*37*). Diastolic blood pressures are reduced by about half as much, but the association increases with age and magnitude of the initial blood pressure. It was estimated that a universal reduction in dietary intake of sodium by 50 mmol per day would lead to a 50% reduction in the number of people requiring antihypertensive therapy, a 22% reduction in the number of deaths resulting from strokes and a 16% reduction in the number of deaths from coronary heart disease. The first prospective study using 24-hour urine collections for measuring sodium intake, which is the only reliable measure, demonstrated a positive relationship between an increased risk of acute coronary events, but not stroke events, and increased sodium excretion (*38*). The association was strongest among overweight men.

Several clinical intervention trials, conducted to evaluate the effects of dietary salt reduction on blood pressure levels, have been systematically reviewed (*39, 40*). Based on an overview of 32 methodologically adequate trials, Cutler, Follmann & Allender (*39*) concluded that a daily reduction of sodium intake by 70–80 mmol was associated with a lowering of blood pressure both in hypertensive and normotensive individuals, with systolic and diastolic blood pressure reductions of 4.8/1.9 mmHg in the former and 2.5/1.1 mmHg in the latter. Clinical trials have also demonstrated the sustainable blood pressure lowering effects of sodium restriction in infancy (*41, 42*), as well as in the elderly in whom it provides a useful non-pharmacological therapy (*43*). The results of a low-sodium diet trial (*44*) showed that low-sodium diets, with 24-hour sodium excretion levels around 70 mmol, are effective and safe. Two population studies, in China and in Portugal, have also revealed significant reductions in blood pressure in the intervention groups (*45, 46*).

A meta-analysis of randomized controlled trials showed that potassium supplements reduced mean blood pressures (systolic/diastolic) by 1.8/1.0 mmHg in normotensive subjects and 4.4/2.5 mmHg in hypertensive subjects (*47*). Several large cohort studies have found an inverse association between potassium intake and risk of stroke (*48, 49*). While potassium supplements have been shown to have protective effects on blood pressure and cardiovascular diseases, there is no evidence to suggest that long-term potassium supplements should be administered to reduce the risk for CVD. The recommended levels of fruit and vegetable consumption assure an adequate intake of potassium.

Food items and food groups
While the consumption of fruits and vegetables has been widely believed to promote good health, evidence related to their protective effect against CVD has only been presented in recent years (*50*). Numerous ecological and prospective studies have reported a significant protective association for coronary heart disease and stroke with consumption of fruits and vegetables (*50–53*). The effects of increased fruit and vegetable consumption on blood pressure alone and in combination with a low-fat diet, were assessed in the Dietary Approaches to Stop Hypertension (DASH) trial (*54*). While the combination diet was more effective in lowering blood pressure, the fruit and vegetable diet also lowered blood pressure (by 2.8 mmHg systolic and 1.1 mmHg diastolic) in comparison to the control diet. Such reductions, while seeming modest at the individual level, would result in a substantial reduction in population-wide risk of CVD by shifting the blood pressure distribution.

Most, but not all, population studies have shown that fish consumption is associated with a reduced risk of coronary heart disease. A systematic review concluded that the discrepancy in the findings may be a result of differences in the populations studied, with only high-risk individuals benefiting from increasing their fish consumption (*55*). It was estimated that in high-risk populations, an optimum fish consumption of 40–60 g per day would lead to approximately a 50% reduction in death from coronary heart disease. In a diet and reinfarction trial, 2-year mortality was reduced by 29% in survivors of a first myocardial infarction in persons receiving advice to consume fatty fish at least twice a week (*56*). A recent study based on data from 36 countries, reported that fish consumption is associated with a reduced risk of death from all causes as well as CVD mortality (*57*).

Several large epidemiological studies have demonstrated that frequent consumption of nuts was associated with decreased risk of coronary heart disease (*58, 59*). Most of these studies considered nuts as a group, combining many different types of nuts. Nuts are high in unsaturated fatty acids and low in saturated fats, and contribute to cholesterol lowering by altering the fatty acid profile of the diet as a whole. However, because of the high energy content of nuts, advice to include them in the diet must be tempered in accordance with the desired energy balance.

Several trials indicate that soy has a beneficial effect on plasma lipids (*60, 61*). A composite analysis of 38 clinical trials found that an average consumption of 47 g of soy protein a day led to a 9% decline in total cholesterol and a 13% decline in LDL cholesterol in subjects free of coronary heart disease (*62*). Soy is rich in isoflavones, compounds that are structurally and functionally similar to estrogen. Several animal experiments suggest that the intake of these isoflavones may provide protection against coronary heart disease, but human data on efficacy and safety are still awaited.

There is convincing evidence that low to moderate alcohol consumption lowers the risk of coronary heart disease. In a systematic review of ecological, case–control and cohort studies in which specific associations were available between risk of coronary heart-disease and consumption of beer, wine and spirits, it was found that all alcoholic drinks are linked with lower risk (*63*). However, other cardiovascular and health risks associated with alcohol do not favour a general recommendation for its use.

Boiled, unfiltered coffee raises total and LDL cholesterol because coffee beans contain a terpenoid lipid called cafestol. The amount of cafestol in the cup depends on the brewing method: it is zero for paper-filtered drip coffee, and high in the unfiltered coffee still widely drunk in, for example, in Greece, the Middle East and Turkey. Intake of large amounts of unfiltered coffee markedly raises serum cholesterol and has been associated with coronary heart disease in Norway (*64*). A shift from unfiltered, boiled coffee to filtered coffee has contributed significantly to the decline in serum cholesterol in Finland (*65*).

5.4.5 *Disease-specific recommendations*

Measures aimed at reducing the risk of CVD are outlined below. The strength of evidence on lifestyle factors is summarized in Table 10.

Fats

Dietary intake of fats strongly influences the risk of cardiovascular diseases such as coronary heart disease and stroke, through effects on blood lipids, thrombosis, blood pressure, arterial (endothelial) function, arrythmogenesis and inflammation. However, the qualitative composition of fats in the diet has a significant role to play in modifying this risk.

Table 10
Summary of strength of evidence on lifestyle factors and risk of developing cardiovascular diseases

Evidence	Decreased risk	No relationship	Increased risk
Convincing	Regular physical activity Linoleic acid Fish and fish oils (EHA and DHA) Vegetables and fruits (including berries) Potassium Low to moderate alcohol intake (for coronary heart disease)	Vitamin E supplements	Myristic and palmitic acids Trans fatty acids High sodium intake Overweight High alcohol intake (for stroke)
Probable	α-Linolenic acid Oleic acid NSP Wholegrain cereals Nuts (unsalted) Plant sterols/stanols Folate	Stearic acid	Dietary cholesterol Unfiltered boiled coffee
Possible	Flavonoids Soy products		Fats rich in lauric acid Impaired fetal nutrition Beta-carotene supplements
Insufficient	Calcium Magnesium Vitamin C		Carbohydrates Iron

EPA, eicosapentaenoic acid; DHA, docosahexaenoic acid; NSP, non-starch polysaccharides.

The evidence shows that intake of saturated fatty acids is directly related to cardiovascular risk. The traditional target is to restrict the intake of saturated fatty acids to less than 10%, of daily energy intake and less than 7% for high-risk groups. If populations are consuming less than 10%, they should not increase that level of intake. Within these limits, intake of foods rich in myristic and palmitic acids should be replaced by fats with a lower content of these particular fatty acids. In developing countries, however, where energy intake for some population groups may be inadequate, energy expenditure is high and body fat stores are low (BMI < 18.5 kg/m²). The amount and quality of fat supply has to be considered keeping in mind the need to meet energy requirements. Specific sources of saturated fat, such as coconut and palm oil, provide low-cost energy and may be an important source of energy for the poor.

Not all saturated fats have similar metabolic effects; those with 12–16 carbons in the fatty acid chain have a greater effect on raising LDL cholesterol. This implies that the fatty acid composition of the fat source should be examined. As populations progress in the nutrition transition and energy excess becomes a potential problem, restricting certain fatty acids becomes progressively more relevant to ensuring cardiovascular health.

To promote cardiovascular health, diets should provide a very low intake of trans fatty acids (hydrogenated oils and fats). In practice, this implies an intake of less than 1% of daily energy intake. This recommendation is especially relevant in developing countries where low-cost hydrogenated fat is frequently consumed. The potential effect of human consumption of hydrogenated oils of unknown physiological effects (e.g. marine oils) is of great concern.

Diets should provide an adequate intake of PUFAs, i.e. in the range 6–10% of daily energy intake. There should also be an optimal balance between intake of n-6 PUFAs and n-3 PUFAs, i.e. 5–8% and 1–2% of daily energy intake, respectively.

Intake of oleic acid, a monounsaturated fatty acid, should make up the rest of the daily energy intake from fats, to give a daily total fat intake ranging from 15% up to 30% of daily energy intake. Recommendations for total fat intake may be based on current levels of population consumption in different regions and modified to take account of age, activity and ideal body weight. Where obesity is prevalent, for example, an intake in the lower part of the range is preferable in order to achieve a lower energy intake. While there is no evidence to directly link the quantity of daily fat intake to an increased risk of CVD, total fat consumption should be limited to enable the goals of reduced intake of saturated and trans fatty acids to be met easily in most populations and to avoid the potential problems of undesirable weight gain that may arise from unrestricted fat intake. It should be noted that highly active groups with diets rich in vegetables, legumes, fruits and wholegrain cereals will limit the risk of unhealthy weight gain on a diet comprising a total fat intake of up to 35%.

These dietary goals can be met by limiting the intake of fat from dairy and meat sources, avoiding the use of hydrogenated oils and fats in cooking and manufacture of food products, using appropriate edible vegetable oils in small amounts, and ensuring a regular intake of fish (one to two times per week) or plant sources of α-linolenic acid. Preference should be given to food preparation practices that employ non-frying methods.

Fruits and vegetables
Fruits and vegetables contribute to cardiovascular health through the variety of phytonutrients, potassium and fibre that they contain. Daily intake of fresh fruit and vegetables (including berries, green leafy and cruciferous vegetables and legumes), in an adequate quantity (400–500 g per day), is recommended to reduce the risk of coronary heart disease, stroke and high blood pressure.

Sodium

Dietary intake of sodium, from all sources, influences blood pressure levels in populations and should be limited so as to reduce the risk of coronary heart disease and both forms of stroke. Current evidence suggests that an intake of no more than 70 mmol or 1.7 g of sodium per day is beneficial in reducing blood pressure. The special situation of individuals (i.e. pregnant women and non-acclimated people who perform strenuous physical activity in hot environments) who may be adversely affected by sodium reduction needs to be kept in mind.

Limitation of dietary sodium intake to meet these goals should be achieved by restricting daily salt (sodium chloride) intake to less than 5 g per day. This should take into account total sodium intake from all dietary sources, for example additives such as monosodium glutamate and preservatives. Use of potassium-enriched low-sodium substitutes is one way to reduce sodium intake. The need to adjust salt iodization, depending on observed sodium intake and surveillance of iodine status of the population, should be recognized.

Potassium

Adequate dietary intake of potassium lowers blood pressure and is protective against stroke and cardiac arrythmias. Potassium intake should be at a level which will keep the sodium to potassium ratio close to 1.0, i.e. a daily potassium intake level of 70–80 mmol per day. This may be achieved through adequate daily consumption of fruits and vegetables.

NSP (dietary fibre)[1]

Fibre is protective against coronary heart disease and has also been used in diets to lower blood pressure. Adequate intake may be achieved through fruits, vegetables and wholegrain cereals.

Fish

Regular fish consumption (1–2 servings per week) is protective against coronary heart disease and ischaemic stroke and is recommended. The serving should provide an equivalent of 200–500 mg of eicosapentaenoic and docosahexaenoic acid. People who are vegetarians are recommended to ensure adequate intake of plant sources of α-linolenic acid.

Alcohol

Although regular low to moderate consumption of alcohol is protective against coronary heart disease, other cardiovascular and health risks associated with alcohol do not favour a general recommendation for its use.

---

[1] Specific amounts will depend on the analytical methodologies used to measure fibre.

Physical activity

Physical activity is related to the risk of cardiovascular diseases, especially coronary heart disease, in a consistent inverse dose–response fashion when either volume or intensity are used for assessment. These relationships apply to both incidence and mortality rates from all cardiovascular diseases and from coronary heart disease. At present, no consistent dose–response relationship can be found between risk of stroke and physical activity. The lower limits of volume or intensity of the protective dose of physical activity have not been defined with certainty, but the current recommendation of at least 30 minutes of at least moderate-intensity physical activity on most days of the week is considered sufficient. A higher volume or intensity of activity would confer a greater protective effect. The recommended amount of physical activity is sufficient to raise cardio-respiratory fitness to the level that has been shown to be related to decreased risk of cardiovascular disease. Individuals who are unaccustomed to regular exercise or have a high-risk profile for CVD should avoid sudden and high-intensity bursts of physical activity.

References

1. Reddy KS. Cardiovascular diseases in the developing countries: dimensions, determinants, dynamics and directions for public health action. *Public Health Nutrition*, 2002, **5**:231–237.

2. Kris-Etherton PM et al. Summary of the scientific conference on dietary fatty acids and cardiovascular health: conference summary from the nutrition committee of the American Heart Association. *Circulation*, 2001, **103**:1034–1039.

3. Grundy SM, Vega GL. Plasma cholesterol responsiveness to saturated fatty acids. *American Journal of Clinical Nutrition*, 1988, **47**:822–824.

4. Katan MJ, Zock PL, Mensink RP. Dietary oils, serum lipoproteins and coronary heart disease. *American Journal of Clinical Nutrition*, 1995, **61**(Suppl. 6):1368–1373.

5. Mensink RP, Katan MB. Effect of dietary fatty acids on serum lipids and lipoproteins. A meta-analysis of 27 trials. *Arteriosclerosis and Thrombosis*, 1992, **12**:911–919.

6. Hu FB et al. Dietary fat intake and the risk of coronary heart disease in women. *New England Journal of Medicine*, 1997, **337**:1491–1499.

7. Katan MB. Trans fatty acids and plasma lipoproteins. *Nutrition Reviews*, 2000, **58**:188–191.

8. Oomen CM et al. Association between trans fatty acid intake and 10-year risk of coronary heart disease in the Zutphen Elderly Study: a prospective population-based study. *Lancet*, 2001, **357**:746–751.

9. Willett WC et al. Intake of trans fatty acids and risk of coronary heart disease among women. *Lancet*, 1993, **341**:581–585.

10. Kris-Etherton PM. Monosaturated fatty acids and risk of cardiovascular disease. *Circulation*, 1999, **100**:1253–1258.

11. Mori TA, Beilin LJ. Long-chain omega 3 fatty acids, blood lipids and cardiovascular risk reduction. *Current Opinion in Lipidology*, 2001, **12**:11–17.

12. GISSI-Prevenzione investigators. Dietary supplementation with n-3 polyunsaturated fatty acids and vitamin E after myocardial infarction: results of the

GISSI-Prevenzione trial. Gruppo Italiano per lo Studio della Sopravvivenza nell'Infarto Miocardico. *Lancet*, 1999, **354**:447–455.

13. **Hu FB et al.** Fish and omega-3 fatty acid intake and risk of coronary heart disease in women. *American Journal of Clinical Nutrition*, 1999, **69**:890–897.

14. **Ascherio A et al.** Dietary fat and risk of coronary heart disease in men: cohort follow-up study in the United States. *British Medical Journal*, 1996, **313**:84–90.

15. **Hopkins PN.** Effects of dietary cholesterol on serum cholesterol: a meta-analysis and review. *American Journal of Clinical Nutrition*, 1992, **55**:1060–1070.

16. **Hu FB et al.** A prospective study of egg consumption and risk of cardiovascular disease in men and women. *Journal of the American Medical Association*, 1999, **281**:1387–1394.

17. **Miettinen TA et al.** Reduction of serum cholesterol with sitostanol-ester margarine in a mildly hypercholesterolemic population. *New England Journal of Medicine*, 1995, **333**:1308–1312.

18. **Law M.** Plant sterols and stanol margarines and health. *British Medical Journal*, 2000, **320**:861–864.

19. **Anderson JW, Hanna TJ.** Impact of nondigestible carbohydrates on serum lipoproteins and risk for cardiovascular disease. *Journal of Nutrition*, 1999, **129**:1457–1466.

20. **Truswell AS.** Cereal grains and coronary heart disease. *European Journal of Clinical Nutrition*, 2002, **56**:1–14.

21. **Liu S et al.** Whole-grain consumption and risk of coronary heart disease: results from the Nurses' Health Study. *American Journal of Clinical Nutrition*, 1999, **70**:412–419.

22. **Pietinen P et al.** Intake of dietary fiber and risk of coronary heart disease in a cohort of Finnish men. The Alpha-Tocopherol, Beta-Carotene Cancer Prevention Study. *Circulation*, 1996, **94**:2720–2727.

23. **Rimm EB et al.** Vegetable, fruit, and cereal fiber intake and risk of coronary heart disease among men. *Journal of the American Medical Association*, 1996, **275**:447–451.

24. **Yusuf S et al.** Vitamin E supplementation and cardiovascular events in high-risk patients. The Heart Outcomes Prevention Evaluation Study Investigators. *New England Journal of Medicine*, 2000, **342**:154–160.

25. **Heart Protection Study Collaborative Group.** MRC/BHF Heart Protection Study of antioxidant vitamin supplementation in 20 536 high-risk individuals: a randomised placebo-controlled trial. *Lancet*, 2002, **360**:23–33.

26. **Egger M, Schneider M, Davey-Smith G.** Spurious precision? Meta-analysis of observational studies. *British Medical Journal*, 1998, **316**:140–144.

27. **Brouwer IA et al.** Low dose folic acid supplementation decreases plasma homocysteine concentrations: a randomized trial. *American Journal of Clinical Nutrition*, 1999, **69**:99–104.

28. **Ueland PM et al.** The controversy over homocysteine and cardiovascular risk. *American Journal of Clinical Nutrition*, 2000, **72**:324–332.

29. **Nygard O et al.** Total plasma homocysteine and cardiovascular risk profile. The Hordaland Homocysteine Study. *Journal of the American Medical Association*, 1995, **274**:1526–1533.

30. **Brattstrom L, Wilcken DEL.** Homocysteine and cardiovascular disease: cause or effect? *American Journal of Clinical Nutrition*, 2000, **72**:315–323.

31. Guttormsen AB et al. Kinetic basis of hyperhomocysteinemia in patients with chronic renal failure. *Kidney International*, 1997, **52**:495–502.

32. Rimm EB et al. Folate and vitamin B6 from diet and supplements in relation to risk of coronary heart disease among women. *Journal of the American Medical Association*, 1998, **279**:359–364.

33. Wald DS, Law M, Morris JK. Homocysteine and cardiovascular disease: evidence on causality from a meta-analysis. *British Medical Journal*, **325**:1202–1208.

34. Keli SO et al. Dietary flavonoids, antioxidant vitamins, and incidence of stroke: the Zutphen study. *Archives of Internal Medicine*, 1996. **156**:637–642.

35. Hertog MGL et al. Dietary antioxidant flavonoids and risk of coronary heart disease: the Zutphen Elderly Study. *Lancet*, 1993, **342**:1007–1011.

36. Gibbs CR, Lip GY, Beevers DG. Salt and cardiovascular disease: clinical and epidemiological evidence. *Journal of Cardiovascular Risk,* 2000, **7**:9–13.

37. Law MR, Frost CD, Wald NJ. By how much does salt reduction lower blood pressure? III–Analysis of data from trials of salt reduction. *British Medical Journal*, 1991, **302**:819–824.

38. Tuomilehto J et al. Urinary sodium excretion and cardiovascular mortality in Finland: a prospective study. *Lancet*, 2001, **357**:848–851.

39. Cutler JA, Follmann D, Allender PS. Randomized trials of sodium reduction: an overview. *American Journal of Clinical Nutrition,* 1997, **65**:643–651.

40. Midgley JP et al. Effect of reduced dietary sodium on blood pressure: a meta-analysis of randomized controlled trials. *Journal of the American Medical Association*, 1996, **275**:1590–1597.

41. Geleijnse JM et al. Long-term effects of neonatal sodium restriction on blood pressure. *Hypertension*, 1997, **29**:913–917 (erratum appears in *Hypertension*, 1997, **29**:1211).

42. Hofman A, Hazebroek A, Valkenburg HA. A randomized trial of sodium intake and blood pressure in newborn infants. *Journal of the American Medical Association*, 1983, **250**:370–373.

43. Whelton PK et al. Sodium reduction and weight loss in the treatment of hypertension in older persons. *Journal of the American Medical Association*, 1998, **279**:839–846 (erratum appears in *Journal of the American Medical Association*, 1998, **279**:1954).

44. Sacks FM et al. Effects on blood pressure of reduced dietary sodium and the Dietary Approaches to Stop Hypertension (DASH) diet. *New England Journal of Medicine*, 2001, **344**:3–10.

45. Forte JG et al. Salt and blood pressure: a community trial. *Journal of Human Hypertension*, 1989, **3**:179–184.

46. Tian HG et al. Changes in sodium intake and blood pressure in a community-based intervention project in China. *Journal of Human Hypertension*, 1995, **9**:959–968.

47. Whelton PK et al. Effects of oral potassium on blood pressure. Meta-analysis of randomized controlled clinical trials. *Journal of the American Medical Association*, 1997, **277**:1624–1632.

48. Ascherio A et al. Intake of potassium, magnesium, and fiber and risk of stroke among US men. *Circulation,* 1998, **98**:1198–1204.

49. Khaw KT, Barrett-Connor E. Dietary potassium and stroke-associated mortality. A 12-year prospective population study. *New England Journal of Medicine*, 1987, 316:235–240.

50. Ness AR, Powles JW. Fruit and vegetables, and cardiovascular disease: a review. *International Journal of Epidemiology*, 1997, 26:1–13.

51. Liu S et al. Fruit and vegetable intake and risk of cardiovascular disease: the Women's Health Study. *American Journal of Clinical Nutrition*, 2000, 72:922–928.

52. Joshipura KJ et al. Fruit and vegetable intake in relation to risk of ischemic stroke. *Journal of the American Medical Association,* 1999, 282:1233–1239.

53. Gilman MW et al. Protective effect of fruits and vegetables on development of stroke in men. *Journal of the American Medical Association*, 1995, 273:1113–1117.

54. Appel LJ et al. A clinical trial of the effects of dietary patterns on blood pressure. DASH Collaborative Research Group. *New England Journal of Medicine,* 1998, 336:1117–1124.

55. Marckmann P, Gronbaek M. Fish consumption and coronary heart disease mortality. A systematic review of prospective cohort studies. *European Journal of Clinical Nutrition*, 1999, 53:585–590.

56. Burr ML et al. Effects of changes in fat, fish and fibre intakes on death and myocardial reinfarction: diet and reinfarction trial (DART). *Lancet,* 1989, 2:757–761.

57. Zhang J et al. Fish consumption and mortality from all causes, ischemic heart disease, and stroke: an ecological study. *Preventive Medicine*, 1999, 28:520–529.

58. Kris-Etherton PM et al. The effects of nuts on coronary heart disease risk. *Nutrition Reviews*, 2001, 59:103–111.

59. Hu FB, Stampfer MJ. Nut consumption and risk of coronary heart disease: a review of epidemiologic evidence. *Current Atherosclerosis Reports,* 1999, 1:204–209.

60. Third International Symposium on the Role of Soy in Preventing and Treating Chronic Disease. *Journal of Nutrition*, 2000, 130(Suppl.):653–711.

61. Crouse JR et al. Randomized trial comparing the effect of casein with that of soy protein containing varying amounts of isoflavones on plasma concentrations of lipids and lipoproteins. *Archives of Internal Medicine*, 1999, 159:2070–2076.

62. Anderson JW, Smith BM, Washnok CS. Cardiovascular and renal benefits of dry bean and soybean intake. *American Journal of Clinical Nutrition*, 1999, 70:464–474.

63. Rimm EB et al. Moderate alcohol intake and lower risk of coronary heart disease: meta-analysis of effects on lipids and haemostatic factors. *British Medical Journal*, 1999, 319:1523–1528.

64. Tverdal A et al. Coffee consumption and death from coronary heart disease in middle-aged Norwegian men and women. *British Medical Journal*, 1990, 300:566–569.

65. Pietinen P et al. Changes in diet in Finland from 1972 to 1992: impact on coronary heart disease risk. *Preventive Medicine*, 1996, 25:243–250.

5.5 Recommendations for preventing cancer

5.5.1 *Background*

Cancer is caused by a variety of identified and unidentified factors. The most important established cause of cancer is tobacco smoking. Other important determinants of cancer risk include diet, alcohol and physical activity, infections, hormonal factors and radiation. The relative importance of cancers as a cause of death is increasing, mostly because of the increasing proportion of people who are old, and also in part because of reductions in mortality from some other causes, especially infectious diseases. The incidence of cancers of the lung, colon and rectum, breast and prostate generally increases in parallel with economic development, while the incidence of stomach cancer usually declines with development.

5.5.2 *Trends*

Cancer is now a major cause of mortality throughout the world and, in the developed world, is generally exceeded only by cardiovascular diseases. An estimated 10 million new cases and over 6 million deaths from cancer occurred in 2000 (*1*). As developing countries become urbanized, patterns of cancer, including those most strongly associated with diet, tend to shift towards those of economically developed countries. Between 2000 and 2020, the total number of cases of cancer in the developing world is predicted to increase by 73% and, in the developed world, to increase by 29%, largely as a result of an increase in the number of old people (*1*).

5.5.3 *Diet, physical activity and cancer*

Dietary factors are estimated to account for approximately 30% of cancers in industrialized countries (*2*), making diet second only to tobacco as a theoretically preventable cause of cancer. This proportion is thought to be about 20% in developing countries (*3*), but may grow with dietary change, particularly if the importance of other causes, especially infections, declines. Cancer rates change as populations move between countries and adopt different dietary (and other) behaviours, further implicating dietary factors in the etiology of cancer.

Body weight and physical inactivity together are estimated to account for approximately one-fifth to one-third of several of the most common cancers, specifically cancers of the breast (postmenopausal), colon, endometrium, kidney and oesophagus (adenocarcinoma) (*4*).

5.5.4 *Strength of evidence*

Research to date has uncovered few definite relationships between diet and cancer risk. Dietary factors for which there is convincing evidence for an increase in risk are overweight and obesity, and a high consumption of alcoholic beverages, aflatoxins, and some forms of salting and fermenting fish. There is also convincing evidence to indicate that physical activity decreases the risk of colon cancer. Factors which probably increase risk include high dietary intake of preserved meats, salt-preserved foods and salt, and very hot (thermally) drinks and food. Probable protective factors are consumption of fruits and vegetables, and physical activity (for breast cancer). After tobacco, overweight and obesity appear to be the most important known avoidable causes of cancer.

The role of diet in the etiology of the major cancers

Cancers of the oral cavity, pharynx and oesophagus. In developed countries the main risk factors for cancers of the oral cavity, pharynx and oesophagus are alcohol and tobacco, and up to 75% of such cancers are attributable to these two lifestyle factors (5). Overweight and obesity are established risk factors specifically for adenocarcinoma (but not squamous cell carcinoma) of the oesophagus (6–8). In developing countries, around 60% of cancers of the oral cavity, pharynx and oesophagus are thought to be a result of micronutrient deficiencies related to a restricted diet that is low in fruits and vegetables and animal products (5, 9). The relative roles of various micronutrients are not yet clear (5, 9). There is also consistent evidence that consuming drinks and foods at a very high temperature increases the risk for these cancers (10). Nasopharyngeal cancer is particularly common in South-East Asia (11), and has been clearly associated with a high intake of Chinese-style salted fish, especially during early childhood (12, 13), as well as with infection with the Epstein-Barr virus (2).

Stomach cancer. Until about 20 years ago stomach cancer was the most common cancer in the world, but mortality rates have been falling in all industrialized countries (14) and stomach cancer is currently much more common in Asia than in North America or Europe (11). Infection with the bacterium *Helicobacter pylori* is an established risk factor, but not a sufficient cause, for the development of stomach cancer (15). Diet is thought to be important in the etiology of this disease; substantial evidence suggests that risk is increased by high intakes of some traditionally preserved salted foods, especially meats and pickles, and with salt per se, and that risk is decreased by high intakes of fruits and vegetables (16), perhaps because of their vitamin C content. Further prospective data are needed, in particular to examine whether some of the dietary associations may be partly confounded by *Helicobacter pylori* infection and whether dietary factors may modify the association of *Helicobacter pylori* with risk.

Colorectal cancer. Colorectal cancer incidence rates are approximately ten-fold higher in developed than in developing countries (11), and it has been suggested that diet-related factors may account for up to 80% of the differences in rates between countries (17). The best established diet-related risk factor is overweight/obesity (8) and physical activity has been consistently associated with a reduced risk of colon cancer (but not of rectal cancer) (8, 18). These factors together, however, do not explain the large variation between populations in colorectal cancer rates. There is almost universal agreement that some aspects of the "westernized" diet are a major determinant of risk; for instance, there is some evidence that risk is increased by high intakes of meat and fat, and that risk is decreased by high intakes of fruits and vegetables, dietary fibre, folate and calcium, but none of these hypotheses has been firmly established.

International correlation studies have shown a strong association between per capita consumption of meat and colorectal cancer mortality (19), and a recent systematic review concluded that preserved meat is associated with an increased risk for colorectal cancer but that fresh meat is not (20). However, most studies have not observed positive associations with poultry or fish (9). Overall, the evidence suggests that high consumption of preserved and red meat probably increases the risk for colorectal cancer.

As with meat, international correlation studies show a strong association between per capita consumption of fat and colorectal cancer mortality (19). However, the results of observational studies of fat and colorectal cancer have, overall, not been supportive of an association with fat intake (9, 21).

Many case–control studies have observed a weak association between the risk of colorectal cancer and high consumption of fruits and vegetables and/or dietary fibre (22, 23), but the results of recent large prospective studies have been inconsistent (24–26). Furthermore, results from randomized controlled trials have not shown that intervention over a 3–4 year period with supplemental fibre or a diet low in fat and high in fibre and fruits and vegetables can reduce the recurrence of colorectal adenomas (27–29). It is possible that some of the inconsistencies are a result of differences between studies in the types of fibre eaten and in the methods for classifying fibre in food tables, or that the association with fruits and vegetables arises principally from an increase in risk at very low levels of consumption (30). On balance, the evidence that is currently available suggests that intake of fruits and vegetables probably reduces the risk for colorectal cancer.

Recent studies have suggested that vitamins and minerals might influence the risk for colorectal cancer. Some prospective studies have suggested that a high intake of folate from diet or vitamin supplements is associated with a reduced risk for colon cancer (31–33). Another promising hypothesis is that relatively high intakes of calcium may reduce the risk for colorectal cancer; several observational studies have supported this hypothesis (9, 34), and two trials have indicated that supplemental calcium may have a modest protective effect on the recurrence of colorectal adenomas (29, 35).

Liver cancer. Approximately 75% of cases of liver cancer occur in developing countries, and liver cancer rates vary over 20-fold between countries, being much higher in sub-Saharan Africa and South-East Asia than in North America and Europe (*11*). The major risk factor for hepatocellular carcinoma, the main type of liver cancer, is chronic infection with hepatitis B, and to a lesser extent, hepatitis C virus (*36*). Ingestion of foods contaminated with the mycotoxin, aflatoxin is an important risk factor among people in developing countries, together with active hepatitis virus infection (*13, 37*). Excessive alcohol consumption is the main diet-related risk factor for liver cancer in industrialized countries, probably via the development of cirrhosis and alcoholic hepatitis (*5*).

Pancreatic cancer. Cancer of the pancreas is more common in industrialized countries than in developing countries (*11, 38*). Overweight and obesity possibly increase the risk (*9, 39*). Some studies have suggested that risk is increased by high intakes of meat, and reduced by high intakes of vegetables, but these data are not consistent (*9*).

Lung cancer. Lung cancer is the most common cancer in the world (*11*). Heavy smoking increases the risk by around 30-fold, and smoking causes over 80% of lung cancers in developed countries (*5*). Numerous observational studies have found that lung cancer patients typically report a lower intake of fruits, vegetables and related nutrients (such as β-carotene) than controls (*9, 34*). The only one of these factors to have been tested in controlled trials, namely β-carotene, has, however, failed to produce any benefit when given as a supplement for up to 12 years (*40–42*). The possible effect of diet on lung cancer risk remains controversial, and the apparent protective effect of fruits and vegetables may be largely the result of residual confounding by smoking, since smokers generally consume less fruit and vegetables than non-smokers. In public health terms, the overriding priority for preventing lung cancer is to reduce the prevalence of smoking.

Breast cancer. Breast cancer is the second most common cancer in the world and the most common cancer among women. Incidence rates are about five times higher in industrialized countries than in less developed countries and Japan (*11*). Much of this international variation is a result of differences in established reproductive risk factors such as age at menarche, parity and age at births, and breastfeeding (*43, 44*), but differences in dietary habits and physical activity may also contribute. In fact, age at menarche is partly determined by dietary factors, in that restricted dietary intake during childhood and adolescence leads to delayed menarche. Adult height, also, is weakly positively associated with risk, and is partly determined by dietary factors during childhood and adolescence (*43*). Estradiol and perhaps other hormones play a key role in the etiology of breast cancer (*43*), and it is possible that any further dietary effects on risk are mediated by hormonal mechanisms.

The only dietary factors which have been shown to increase the risk for breast cancer are obesity and alcohol. Obesity increases breast cancer risk in postmenopausal women by around 50%, probably by increasing serum concentrations of free estradiol (*43*). Obesity does not increase risk among premenopausal women, but obesity in premenopausal women is likely to lead to obesity throughout life and therefore to an eventual increase in breast cancer risk. For alcohol, there is now a large body of data from well-designed studies which consistently shows a small increase in risk with increasing consumption, with about a 10% increase in risk for an average of one alcoholic drink every day (*45*). The mechanism for this association is not known, but may involve increases in estrogen levels (*46*).

The results of studies of other dietary factors including fat, meat, dairy products, fruits and vegetables, fibre and phyto-estrogens are inconclusive (*9, 34, 47, 48*).

Endometrial cancer. Endometrial cancer risk is about three-fold higher in obese women than in lean women (*8, 49*), probably because of the effects of obesity on hormone levels (*50*). Some case–control studies have suggested that diets high in fruits and vegetables may reduce risk and that diets high in saturated or total fat may increase risk, but the amount of available data is limited (*9*).

Prostate cancer. Prostate cancer incidence rates are strongly affected by diagnostic practices and therefore difficult to interpret, but mortality rates show that death from prostate cancer is about 10 times more common in North America and Europe than in Asia (*11*).

Little is known about the etiology of prostate cancer, although ecological studies suggest that it is positively associated with a "westernized" diet (*19*). The data from prospective studies have not established causal or protective associations for specific nutrients or dietary factors (*9, 34*). Diets high in red meat, dairy products and animal fat have frequently been implicated in the development of prostate cancer, although the data are not entirely consistent (*9, 51–53*). Randomized controlled trials have provided substantial, consistent evidence that supplements of β-carotene do not alter the risk for prostate cancer (*40, 41, 54*) but have suggested that vitamin E (*54*) and selenium (*55*) might have a protective effect. Lycopene, primarily from tomatoes, has been associated with a reduced risk in some observational studies, but the data are not consistent (*56*). Hormones control the growth of the prostate, and diet might influence prostate cancer risk by affecting hormone levels.

Kidney cancer. Overweight and obesity are established risk factors for cancer of the kidney, and may account for up to 30% of kidney cancers in both men and women (*57*).

Table 11 provides a summary of strength of evidence with regard to the role of various risk factors in the development of cancer.

Table 11
Summary of strength of evidence on lifestyle factors and the risk of developing cancer

Evidence	Decreased risk	Increased risk
Convincing[a]	Physical activity (colon)	Overweight and obesity (oesophagus, colorectum, breast in postmenopausal women, endometrium, kidney)
		Alcohol (oral cavity, pharynx, larynx, oesophagus, liver, breast)
		Aflatoxin (liver)
		Chinese-style salted fish (nasopharynx)
Probable[a]	Fruits and vegetables (oral cavity, oesophagus, stomach, colorectum[b])	Preserved meat (colorectum)
		Salt-preserved foods and salt (stomach)
	Physical activity (breast)	Very hot (thermally) drinks and food (oral cavity, pharynx, oesophagus)
Possible/ insufficient	Fibre	Animal fats
	Soya	Heterocyclic amines
	Fish	Polycyclic aromatic hydrocarbons
	n-3 Fatty acids	Nitrosamines
	Carotenoids	
	Vitamins B_2, B_6, folate, B_{12}, C, D, E	
	Calcium, zinc and selenium	
	Non-nutrient plant constituents (e.g. allium compounds, flavonoids, isoflavones, lignans)	

[a] The "convincing" and "probable" categories in this report correspond to the "sufficient" category of the IARC report on weight control and physical activity (*4*) in terms of the public health and policy implications.
[b] For colorectal cancer, a protective effect of fruit and vegetable intake has been suggested by many case–control studies but this has not been supported by results of several large prospective studies, suggesting that if a benefit does exist it is likely to be modest.

The Consultation recognized the problems posed by the lack of data on diet and cancer from the developing world. There are very limited data from Africa, Asia and Latin America, yet these regions represent two-thirds or more of the world population. There is thus an urgent need for epidemiological research on diet and cancer in these regions. The need to evaluate the role of food processing methods, traditional and industrial, was also identified. Microbiological and chemical food contaminants may also contribute to carcinogenicity of diets.

The nutrition transition is accompanied by changes in prevalence of specific cancers. For some cancers, such as stomach cancer, this may be beneficial while for others, such as colorectal and breast cancers, the changes are adverse.

5.5.5 *Disease-specific recommendations*

The main recommendations for reducing the risk of developing cancer are as follows:

- Maintain weight (among adults) such that BMI is in the range of 18.5–24.9 kg/m^2 and avoid weight gain (> 5 kg) during adult life (*58*).
- Maintain regular physical activity. The primary goal should be to perform physical activity on most days of the week; 60 minutes per day of moderate-intensity activity, such as walking, may be needed to maintain healthy body weight in otherwise sedentary people. More vigorous activity, such as fast walking, may give some additional benefits for cancer prevention (*4*).
- Consumption of alcoholic beverages is not recommended: if consumed, do not exceed two units[1] per day.
- Chinese-style fermented salted fish should only be consumed in moderation, especially during childhood. Overall consumption of salt-preserved foods and salt should be moderate.
- Minimize exposure to aflatoxin in foods.
- Have a diet which includes at least 400 g per day of total fruits and vegetables.
- Those who are not vegetarian are advised to moderate consumption of preserved meat (e.g. sausages, salami, bacon, ham).[2]
- Do not consume foods or drinks when they are at a very hot (scalding hot) temperature.

References

1. Parkin DM. Global cancer statistics in the year 2000. *Lancet Oncology*, 2001, 2:533–543.

2. Doll R, Peto R. Epidemiology of cancer. In: Weatherall DJ, Ledingham JGG, Warrell DA, eds. *Oxford textbook of medicine*. Oxford, Oxford University Press, 1996:197–221.

3. Willet MC. Diet, nutrition, and avoidable cancer. *Environmental Health Perspectives*, 1995, **103**(Suppl. 8):S165–S170.

4. *Weight control and physical activity*. Lyon, International Agency for Research on Cancer, 2002 (IARC Handbooks of Cancer Prevention, Vol. 6).

5. *Cancer: causes, occurrence and control*. Lyon, International Agency for Research on Cancer, 1990 (IARC Scientific Publications, No. 100).

6. Brown LM et al. Adenocarcinoma of the esophagus: role of obesity and diet. *Journal of the National Cancer Institute*, 1995, **87**:104–109.

7. Cheng KK et al. A case–control study of oesophageal adenocarcinoma in women: a preventable disease. *British Journal of Cancer*, 2000, **83**:127–132.

---

[1] One unit is equivalent to approximately 10 g of alcohol and is provided by one glass of beer, wine or spirits.

[2] Poultry and fish (except Chinese-style salted fish) have been studied and found not to be associated with increased risk for cancer.

8. Overweight and lack of exercise linked to increased cancer risk. In: *Weight control and physical activity*. Lyon, International Agency for Research on Cancer, 2002 (IARC Handbooks of Cancer Prevention, Vol. 6).

9. *Food, nutrition and the prevention of cancer: a global perspective*. Washington, DC, World Cancer Research Fund/American Institute for Cancer Research, 1997.

10. Sharp L et al. Risk factors for squamous cell carcinoma of the oesophagus in women: a case–control study. *British Journal of Cancer*, 2001, **85**:1667–1670.

11. Ferlay J et al. *Globocan 2000: cancer incidence, mortality and prevalence worldwide*. Version 1.0. Lyon, International Agency for Research on Cancer, 2001 (IARC CancerBase No. 5; available on the Internet at http://www-dep.iarc.fr/globocan/globocan.html).

12. Yu MC. Nasopharyngeal carcinoma: epidemiology and dietary factors. In: O'Neill IK, Chen J, Bartsch H, eds. *Relevance to human cancer of N-nitroso compounds, tobacco smoke and mycotoxins*. Lyon, International Agency for Research on Cancer, 1991:39–47 (IARC Scientific Publications, No. 105).

13. *Some naturally occurring substances: food items and constituents, heterocyclic aromatic amines and mycotoxins*. Lyon, International Agency for Research on Cancer, 1993 (IARC Monographs on the Evaluation of Carcinogenic Risks to Humans, Vol. 56).

14. *World health statistics annual*. Geneva, World Health Organization, 2001 (available on the Internet at http://www.who.int/whosis/).

15. Helicobacter and Cancer Collaborative Group. Gastric cancer and *Helicobacter pylori*: a combined analysis of 12 case–control studies nested within prospective cohorts. *Gut*, 2001, **49**:347–353.

16. Palli D. Epidemiology of gastric cancer: an evaluation of available evidence. *Journal of Gastroenterology*, 2000, **35**(Suppl. 12):S84–S89.

17. Cummings JH, Bingham SA. Diet and the prevention of cancer. *British Medical Journal*, 1998, **317**:1636–1640.

18. Hardman AE. Physical activity and cancer risk. *Proceedings of the Nutrition Society*, 2001, **60**:107–113.

19. Armstrong B, Doll R. Environmental factors and cancer incidence and mortality in different countries, with special reference to dietary practices. *International Journal of Cancer*, 1975, **15**:617–631.

20. Norat T et al. Meat consumption and colorectal cancer risk: a dose–response meta-analysis of epidemiological studies. *International Journal of Cancer*, 2002, **98**:241–256.

21. Howe GR et al. The relationship between dietary fat intake and risk of colorectal cancer: evidence from the combined analysis of 13 case–control studies. *Cancer Causes and Control*, 1997, **8**:215–228.

22. Potter JD, Steinmetz K. Vegetables, fruit and phytoestrogens as preventive agents. In: Stewart BW, McGregor D, Kleihues P, eds. *Principles of chemoprevention*. Lyon, International Agency for Research on Cancer, 1996:61–90 (IARC Scientific Publications, No. 139).

23. Jacobs DR Jr et al. Whole-grain intake and cancer: an expanded review and meta-analysis. *Nutrition and Cancer*, 1998, **30**:85–96.

24. Bueno de Mesquita HB, Ferrari P, Riboli E (on behalf of EPIC Working Group on Dietary Patterns). Plant foods and the risk of colorectal cancer in Europe: preliminary findings. In: Riboli E, Lambert R, eds. *Nutrition and lifestyle:*

opportunities for cancer prevention. Lyon, International Agency for Research on Cancer, 2002:89–95 (IARC Scientific Publications, No. 156).

25. **Fuchs CS et al.** Dietary fiber and the risk of colorectal cancer and adenoma in women. *New England Journal of Medicine,* 1999, **340**:169–176.

26. **Michels KB et al.** Prospective study of fruit and vegetable consumption and incidence of colon and rectal cancers. *Journal of the National Cancer Institute,* 2000, **92**:1740–1752.

27. **Schatzkin A et al.** Lack of effect of a low-fat, high-fiber diet on the recurrence of colorectal adenomas. Polyp Prevention Trial Study Group. *New England Journal of Medicine,* 2000, **342**:1149–1155.

28. **Alberts DS et al.** Lack of effect of a high-fiber cereal supplement on the recurrence of colorectal adenomas. Phoenix Colon Cancer Prevention Physicians' Network. *New England Journal of Medicine,* 2000, **342**:1156–1162.

29. **Bonithon-Kopp C et al.** Calcium and fibre supplementation in prevention of colorectal adenoma recurrence: a randomised intervention trial. European Cancer Prevention Organisation Study Group. *Lancet,* 2000, **356**:1300–1306.

30. **Terry P et al.** Fruit, vegetables, dietary fiber, and risk of colorectal cancer. *Journal of the National Cancer Institute,* 2001, **93**:525–533.

31. **Giovannucci E et al.** Alcohol, low-methionine, low-folate diets, and risk of colon cancer in men. *Journal of the National Cancer Institute,* 1995, **87**:265–273.

32. **Glynn SA et al.** Alcohol consumption and risk of colorectal cancer in a cohort of Finnish men. *Cancer Causes and Control,* 1996, **7**:214–223.

33. **Giovannucci E et al.** Multivitamin use, folate, and colon cancer in women in the Nurses' Health Study. *Annals of Internal Medicine,* 1998, **129**:517–524.

34. *Nutritional Aspects of the Development of Cancer. Report of the Working Group on Diet and Cancer of the Committee on Medical Aspects of Food and Nutrition Policy.* London, The Stationery Office, 1998 (Report on Health and Social Subjects, No. 48).

35. **Baron JA et al.** Calcium supplements and colorectal adenomas. Polyp Prevention Trial Study Group. *Annals of the New York Academy of Sciences,* 1999, **889**:138–145.

36. *Hepatitis viruses.* Lyon, International Agency for Research on Cancer, 1994 (IARC Monographs on the Evaluation of Carcinogenic Risks to Humans, Vol. 59).

37. **Saracco G.** Primary liver cancer is of multifactorial origin: importance of hepatitis B virus infection and dietary aflatoxin. *Journal of Gastroenterology and Hepatology,* 1995, **10**:604–608.

38. **Parkin DM et al.** Estimating the world cancer burden: globocan 2000. *International Journal of Cancer,* 2001, **94**:153–156.

39. **Michaud DS et al.** Physical activity, obesity, height, and the risk of pancreatic cancer. *Journal of the American Medical Association,* 2001, **286**:921–929.

40. **Hennekens CH et al.** Lack of effect of long-term supplementation with beta-carotene on the incidence of malignant neoplasms and cardiovascular disease. *New England Journal of Medicine,* 1996, **334**:1145–1149.

41. **Omenn GS et al.** Effects of a combination of beta carotene and vitamin A on lung cancer and cardiovascular disease. *New England Journal of Medicine,* 1996, **334**:1150–1155.

42. Beta Carotene Cancer Prevention Study Group The Alpha-Tocopherol. The effect of vitamin E and beta carotene on the incidence of lung cancer and other cancers in male smokers. *New England Journal of Medicine,* 1994, 330:1029–1035.

43. Key TJ, Verkasalo PK, Banks E. Epidemiology of breast cancer. *Lancet Oncology,* 2001, 2:133–140.

44. Collaborative Group on Hormonal Factors in Breast Cancer. Breast cancer and breastfeeding: collaborative reanalysis of individual data from 47 epidemiological studies in 30 countries, including 50 302 women with breast cancer and 96 973 women without the disease. *Lancet,* 2002, 360:187–195.

45. Smith-Warner SA et al. Alcohol and breast cancer in women: a pooled analysis of cohort studies. *Journal of the American Medical Association,* 1998, 279:535–540.

46. Dorgan JF et al. Serum hormones and the alcohol–breast cancer association in postmenopausal women. *Journal of the National Cancer Institute,* 2001, 93:710–715.

47. Key TJ, Allen NE. Nutrition and breast cancer. *Breast,* 2001, 10(Suppl. 3):S9–S13.

48. Smith-Warner SA et al. Intake of fruits and vegetables and risk of breast cancer: a pooled analysis of cohort studies. *Journal of the American Medical Association,* 2001, 285:769–776.

49. Bergstrom A et al. Overweight as an avoidable cause of cancer in Europe. *International Journal of Cancer,* 2001, 91:421–430.

50. Key TJ, Pike MC. The dose–effect relationship between "unopposed" oestrogens and endometrial mitotic rate: its central role in explaining and predicting endometrial cancer risk. *British Journal of Cancer,* 1988, 57:205–212.

51. Schuurman AG et al. Animal products, calcium and protein and prostate cancer risk in The Netherlands Cohort Study. *British Journal of Cancer,* 1999, 80:1107–1113.

52. Chan JM et al. Dairy products, calcium, and prostate cancer risk in the Physicians' Health Study. *American Journal of Clinical Nutrition,* 2001, 74:549–554.

53. Michaud DS et al. A prospective study on intake of animal products and risk of prostate cancer. *Cancer Causes and Control,* 2001, 12:557–567.

54. Heinonen OP et al. Prostate cancer and supplementation with alpha-tocopherol and beta-carotene: incidence and mortality in a controlled trial. *Journal of the National Cancer Institute,* 1998, 90:440–446.

55. Clark LC et al. Decreased incidence of prostate cancer with selenium supplementation: results of a double-blind cancer prevention trial. *British Journal of Urology,* 1998, 81:730–734.

56. Kristal AR, Cohen JH. Invited commentary: tomatoes, lycopene, and prostate cancer. How strong is the evidence? *American Journal of Epidemiology,* 2000, 151:124–127.

57. Bergstrom A et al. Obesity and renal cell cancer—a quantitative review. *British Journal of Cancer,* 2001, 85:984–990.

58. *Obesity: preventing and managing the global epidemic. Report of a WHO Consultation.* Geneva, World Health Organization, 2000 (WHO Technical Report Series, No. 894).

5.6 Recommendations for preventing dental diseases

5.6.1 *Background*

Oral health is related to diet in many ways, for example, through nutritional influences on cranio-facial development, oral cancer and oral infectious diseases. The purpose of this review, however, is to focus on the nutritional aspects of dental diseases. Dental diseases include dental caries, developmental defects of enamel, dental erosion and periodontal disease. Dental diseases are a costly burden to health care services, accounting for between 5% and 10% of total health care expenditures and exceeding the cost of treating cardiovascular disease, cancer and osteoporosis in industrialized countries (*1*). In low-income countries, the cost of traditional restorative treatment of dental disease would probably exceed the available resources for health care. Dental health promotion and preventive strategies are clearly more affordable and sustainable.

Although not life-threatening, dental diseases have a detrimental effect on quality of life in childhood through to old age, having an impact on self-esteem, eating ability, nutrition and health. In modern society, a significant role of teeth is to enhance appearance; facial appearance is very important in determining an individual's integration into society, and teeth also play an essential role in speech and communication. Oral diseases are associated with considerable pain, anxiety and impaired social functioning (*2, 3*). Dental decay may result in tooth loss, which reduces the ability to eat a nutritious diet, the enjoyment of food, the confidence to socialize and the quality of life (*4–6*).

5.6.2 *Trends*

The amount of dental decay is measured using the dmf/DMF index, a count of the number of teeth or surfaces in a person's mouth that are decayed, missing or filled as a result of caries in primary dentition/ permanent dentition. An additional dental status indicator is the proportion of the population who are edentulous (have no natural teeth).

In most low-income countries, the prevalence rate of dental caries is relatively low and more than 90% of caries are untreated. Available data (*7*) show that the mean number of decayed, missing or filled permanent teeth (DMFT) at age 12 years in low-income countries is 1.9, 3.3 in middle-income countries and 2.1 in high-income countries (Table 12).

Data on the level of dental caries in the permanent dentition of 12-year-olds show two distinct trends. First, a fall in the prevalence of dental caries in developed countries, and second an increase in the prevalence of the disease in some developing countries that have increased their consumption of sugars and have not yet been introduced to the presence of adequate amounts of fluoride. Despite the marked overall decline in dental caries over the past 30 years, the prevalence of dental caries remains unacceptably high in many developed countries. Even in countries with low average DMFT scores, a significant proportion of children have relatively high levels of dental caries. Moreover, there is some indication that the favourable trends in levels of dental caries in permanent teeth have come to a halt (8).

Table 12
Trends in levels of dental caries in 12-year-olds (mean DMFT per person aged 12 years)

Country or area	Year	DMFT	Year	DMFT	Year	DMFT
Industrialized countries						
Australia	1956	9.3	1982	2.1	1998	0.8
Finland	1975	7.5	1982	4.0	1997	1.1
Japan	1975	5.9	1993	3.6	1999	2.4
Norway	1940	12.0	1979	4.5	1999	1.5
Romania	1985	5.0	1991	4.3	1996	3.8
Switzerland	1961–1963	9.6	1980	1.7	1996	0.8
United Kingdom	1983	3.1	1993	1.4	1996–1997	1.1
United States	1946	7.6	1980	2.6	1998	1.4
Developing countries						
Chile	1960	2.8	1978	6.6	1996	4.1
Democratic Republic of the Congo	1971	0.1	1982	0.3	1987	0.4–1.1
French Polynesia	1966	6.5	1986	3.2	1994	3.2
Islamic Republic of Iran	1974	2.4	1976	4.9	1995	2.0
Jordan	1962	0.2	1981	2.7	1995	3.3
Mexico	1975	5.3	1991	2.5–5.1	1997	2.5
Morocco	1970	2.6	1980	4.5	1999	2.5
Philippines	1967	1.4	1981	2.9	1998	4.6
Uganda	1966	0.4	1987	0.5	1993	0.4

DMFT, decayed, missing, filled permanent teeth.
Source: reference 7.

Many developing countries have low decayed, missing, filled primary teeth (dmft) values but a high prevalence of dental caries in the primary dentition. Data on 5-year-old children in Europe suggest that the trend towards reduced prevalence of dental decay has halted (9–11). In children aged 5–7 years, average dmft values of below 2.0 have been reported for Denmark, England, Finland, Italy, Netherlands and Norway (12). Higher dmft values were reported recently for Belarus (4.7) (13), Hungary (4.5) (14), Romania (4.3) (15) and the Russian Federation (4.7) (16).

Being free from caries at age 12 years does not imply being caries-free for life. The mean DMFT in countries of the European Union after 1988 varied between 13.4 and 20.8 at 35–44 years (17). The WHO guidelines on oral health state that at age 35–44 years a DMFT score of 14 or above is considered high. In most developing countries, the level of caries in adults of this age group is lower, for example, 2.1 in China (*18*) and 5.7 in Niger (*19*). Few data are available on the prevalence and severity of root caries in older adults, but with the increasingly ageing population and greater retention of teeth, the problem of root caries is likely to become a significant public health concern in the future.

The number of edentulous persons has declined over the past 20–30 years in several industrialized countries (*3*). Despite overall gains however, there is still a large proportion of older adults who are edentulous or partially dentate and as the population continues to age tooth loss will affect a growing number of persons worldwide. Table 13 summarizes the available information on the prevalence of edentulousness in old-age populations throughout the world.

Dental erosion is a relatively new dental problem in many countries throughout the world, and is related to diet. There is anecdotal evidence that prevalence is increasing in industrialized countries, but there are no data over time to indicate patterns of this disease. There are insufficient data available to comment on worldwide trends; in some populations, however, it is thought that approximately 50% of children are affected (*20*).

5.6.3 *Diet and dental disease*

Nutritional status affects the teeth pre-eruptively, although this influence is much less important than the post-eruptive local effect of diet on the teeth (*21*). Deficiencies of vitamins D and A and protein–energy malnutrition have been associated with enamel hypoplasia and salivary gland atrophy (which reduces the mouth's ability to buffer plaque acids), which render the teeth more susceptible to decay. In developing countries, in the absence of dietary sugars, undernutrition is not associated with dental caries. Undernutrition coupled with a high intake of sugars may exacerbate the risk of caries.

There is some evidence to suggest that periodontal disease progresses more rapidly in undernourished populations (*22*); the important role of nutrition in maintaining an adequate host immune response may explain this observation. Apart from severe vitamin C deficiency, which may result in scurvy-related periodontitis, there is little evidence at present for an association between diet and periodontal disease. Current research is investigating the potential role of the antioxidant nutrients in periodontal disease. Poor oral hygiene is the most important risk factor in the development of periodontal disease (*21*). Undernutrition exacerbates the severity of oral infections (e.g. acute necrotizing ulcerative gingivitis) and may eventually lead to their evolution into life-threatening diseases such as noma, a dehumanizing oro-facial gangrene (*23*).

Table 13
Prevalence of edentulousness in older people throughout the world

Country or area	Prevalence of edentulousness (%)	Age group (years)
African Region		
Gambia	6	65 +
Madagascar	25	65–74
Region of the Americas		
Canada	58	65 +
United Sates	26	65–69
South-East Asian Region		
India	19	65–74
Indonesia	24	65 +
Sri Lanka	37	65–74
Thailand	16	65 +
European Region		
Albania	69	65 +
Austria	15	65–74
Bosnia and Herzegovina	78	65 +
Bulgaria	53	65 +
Denmark	27	65–74
Finland	41	65 +
Hungary	27	65–74
Iceland	15	65–74
Italy	19	65–74
Lithuania	14	65–74
Poland	25	65–74
Romania	26	65–74
Slovakia	44	65–74
Slovenia	16	65 +
United Kingdom	46	65 +
Eastern Mediterranean Region		
Egypt	7	65 +
Lebanon	20	64–75
Saudi Arabia	31–46	65 +
Western Pacific Region		
Cambodia	13	65–74
China	11	65–74
Malaysia	57	65 +
Singapore	21	65 +

Source: reference 7.

Dental caries occur because of demineralization of enamel and dentine by organic acids formed by bacteria in dental plaque through the anaerobic metabolism of sugars derived from the diet (24). Organic acids increase the solubility of calcium hydroxyapatite in the dental hard tissues and demineralization occurs. Saliva is super-saturated with calcium and phosphate at pH 7 which promotes remineralization. If the oral pH remains high enough for sufficient time then complete remineralization of enamel may occur. If the acid challenge is too great, however, demineralization dominates and the enamel becomes more porous until finally a carious lesion forms (25). The development of caries requires the presence of sugars and bacteria, but is influenced by the susceptibility of the tooth, the bacterial profile, and the quantity and quality of the saliva.

Dietary sugars and dental caries

There is a wealth of evidence from many different types of investigation, including human studies, animal experiments and experimental studies in vivo and in vitro to show the role of dietary sugars in the etiology of dental caries (21). Collectively, data from these studies provide an overall picture of the cariogenic potential of carbohydrates. Sugars are undoubtedly the most important dietary factor in the development of dental caries. Here, the term "sugars" refers to all monosaccharides and disaccharides, while the term "sugar" refers only to sucrose. The term "free sugars" refers to all monosaccharides and disaccharides added to foods by the manufacturer, cook or consumer, plus sugars naturally present in honey, fruit juices and syrups. The term "fermentable carbohydrate" refers to free sugars, glucose polymers, oligosaccharides and highly refined starches; it excludes non-starch polysaccharides and raw starches.

Worldwide epidemiological studies have compared sugar consumption and levels of dental caries at the between-country level. Sreebny (26, 27) correlated the dental caries experience (DMFT) of 12-year-olds with data on sugar supplies of 47 countries and found a significant correlation ($+0.7$); 52% of the variation in the level of caries was explained by the per capita availability of sugar. In countries with a consumption level of sugar <18 kg per person per year caries experience was consistently $<$ DMFT 3. A later analysis by Woodward & Walker (28) did not find a similar association for developed countries. Sugar availability nevertheless accounted for 28% of the variation in levels of dental caries; 23 out of 26 countries with a per capita sugar availability <50 g per day had a mean DMFT score for 12-year olds of <3, whereas only half of the countries with sugar availability above this level had achieved a DMFT score that was <3.

Miyazaki & Morimoto (29) reported a significant correlation ($r = +0.91$) between sugar availability in Japan and DMFT at age 12 years between 1957 and 1987. Populations that had experienced a reduced sugar availability during the Second World War showed a reduction in dental caries which subsequently increased again when the restriction was lifted (30–32). Although the data pre-date the widespread use of fluoride dentifrice, Weaver (33) observed a reduction in dental caries between 1943 and 1949 in areas of northern England with both high and low concentrations of fluoride in drinking-water.

Isolated communities with a traditional way of life and a consistently low intake of sugars have very low levels of dental caries. As economic levels in such societies rise, the amount of sugar and other fermentable carbohydrates in the diet increases and this is often associated with a marked increase in dental caries. Examples of this trend have been reported among the Inuit in Alaska, USA (34), as well as in populations in Ethiopia (35), Ghana (36), Nigeria (37), Sudan (38), and on the Island of Tristan da Cunha, St Helena (39).

There is evidence to show that many groups of people with high exposure to sugars have levels of caries higher than the population average. Examples include children with chronic diseases requiring long-term sugar-containing medicines (40), and confectionery workers (41–44). Likewise, experience of dental caries has seldom been reported in groups of people who have a habitually low intake of sugars, for example, children of dentists (45, 46) and children in institutions where strict dietary regimens are inflicted (47, 48). A weakness of population studies of this type is that changes in intake of sugars often occur concurrently with changes in the intake of refined starches, making it impossible to attribute changes in dental caries solely to changes in the intake of sugars. An exception to this are the data from studies of children with hereditary fructose intolerance (HFI). Studies have shown that people with HFI have a low intake of sugars and a higher than average intake of starch, but have a low dental caries experience (49).

Human intervention studies are rare, and those that have been reported are now decades old and were conducted in the pre-fluoride era before the strong link between sugars intake and dental caries levels was established. It would not be possible to repeat such studies today because of ethical constraints. The Vipeholm study, conducted in an adult mental institution in Sweden between 1945 and 1953 (50), investigated the effects of consuming sugary foods of varying stickiness and at different times throughout the day on the development of caries. It was found that sugar, even when consumed in large amounts, had little effect on caries increment if it was ingested up to a maximum of four times a day at mealtimes only. Increased frequency of consumption of sugar between meals was, however, associated with a marked increase in dental caries. It was also found that the increase in dental caries activity disappears on withdrawal of sugar-rich foods. Despite the complicated nature of the study the conclusions are valid, although they apply to the pre-fluoride era. The Turku study was a controlled dietary intervention study carried out on adults in Finland in the 1970s which showed that almost total substitution of sucrose in the diet with xylitol (a non-cariogenic sweetener) resulted in an 85% reduction in dental caries over a 2-year period (51).

Numerous cross-sectional epidemiological studies have compared sugars intake with dental caries levels in many countries of the world. Those conducted before the early 1990s have been summarized by Rugg-Gunn (*21*). Nine out of 21 studies that compared amount of sugars consumed with caries increment found significant associations, while the other 12 did not. Moreover, 23 out of 37 studies that investigated the association between frequency of sugars consumption and caries levels found significant relationships, while 14 failed to find any such associations.

A cross-sectional study in the United States of 2514 people aged 9–29 years conducted between 1968 and 1970 found that the dental caries experience of adolescents eating the highest amounts of sugars (upper 15% of the sample) was twice that of those eating the lowest amounts (lower 15% of the sample) (*52*). Granath et al. (*53*) showed that intake of sugars was the most important factor associated with caries in the primary dentition of preschool children in Sweden. When the effects of oral hygiene and fluoride were kept constant, the children with a low intake of sugars between meals had up to 86% less caries than those with high intakes of sugars. Other studies have found fluoride exposure and oral hygiene to be more strongly associated with caries than sugars consumption (*54, 55*). A recent study in the United Kingdom of a representative sample of children aged 4–18 years showed no significant relationship between caries experience and level of intake of free sugars; in the age group 15–18 years, however, the upper band of free sugars consumers were more likely to have decay than the lower band (70% compared with 52%) (*20*).

Many other cross-sectional studies have shown a relationship between sugars consumption and levels of caries in the primary and/or permanent dentitions in countries or areas throughout the world, including China (*56*), Denmark (57), Madagascar (*58, 59*), Saudi Arabia (*60*), Sweden (*61, 62*), Thailand (*63*) and the United Kingdom (*64*).

When investigating the association between diet and the development of dental caries it is more appropriate to use a longitudinal study design in which sugars consumption habits over time are related to changes in dental caries experience. Such studies have shown a significant relationship between caries development and sugars intake (*65–67*). In a comprehensive study of over 400 children in England aged 11–12 years, a small but significant relationship was found between intake of total sugars and caries increment over 2 years ($r = +0.2$) (*67*). The Michigan Study in the United States investigated the relationship between sugars intake and dental caries increment over 3 years in children initially aged 10–15 years (*66*). A weak relationship was found between the amount of dietary sugars consumed and dental caries experience.

In a review of longitudinal studies, Marthaler (68) analysed the relationship between dietary sugars and caries activity in countries where the availability of sugars is high and the use of fluoride is extensive. He concluded that in modern societies that make use of prevention, the relationship between sugars consumption and dental caries was still evident (68). He also concluded that many older studies had failed to show a relationship between sugars intake and development of dental caries because they were of poor methodological design, used unsuitable methods of dietary analysis or were of insufficient power (68). Correlations between individuals' sugars consumption and dental caries increments may be weak if the range of sugars intake in the study population is small. That is to say, that if all people within a population are exposed to the disease risk factor, the relationship between the risk factor and the disease will not be apparent (69).

Frequency and amount of sugars consumption. Several studies, including the above-mentioned Vipeholm study in Sweden, have indicated that caries experience increases markedly when the frequency of sugars intake exceeds four times a day (50, 70–72). The importance of frequency versus the total amount of sugars is difficult to evaluate as the two variables are hard to distinguish from each other. Data from animal studies have indicated the importance of frequency of sugars intake in the development of dental caries (73, 74). Some human studies have also shown that the frequency of sugars intake is an important etiological factor for caries development (75). Many studies have related the frequency of intake of sugars or sugars-rich food to caries development but have not simultaneously investigated the relationship between amount of sugars consumed and dental caries, and therefore no conclusion regarding the relative importance of these two variables can be drawn from these studies (76–78).

Animal studies have also shown a relationship between amount of sugars consumed and the development of dental caries (79–82). Several longitudinal studies in humans have indicated that the amount of sugars consumed is more important than the frequency (66, 67, 83, 84), while Jamel et al. (85) found that both the frequency and the amount of sugars intake are important.

The strong correlation between both the amount and frequency of sugars consumption has been demonstrated by several investigators in different countries (67, 86–88). It is therefore highly likely that, in terms of caries development, both variables are potentially important.

Relative cariogenicity of different sugars and food consistency. The relative acidogenicity of different monosaccharides and disaccharides has been investigated in plaque pH studies, which have shown that lactose is less acidogenic than other sugars (89). Animal studies have provided no clear evidence that, with the exception of lactose, the cariogenicity of monosaccharides and disaccharides differs. The above-mentioned study in Turku, Finland, found no difference in caries development between subjects on diets sweetened with sucrose compared with those whose diet had been sweetened with fructose (51). Invert sugar (50% fructose + 50% glucose) is less cariogenic than sucrose (90).

The adhesiveness or stickiness of a food is not necessarily related to either oral retention time or cariogenic potential. For example, consumption of sugars-containing drinks (i.e. non-sticky) is associated with increased risk of dental caries (85, 88)

Potential impact of sugars reduction on other dietary components. It is important to consider the potential impact of a reduction in free sugars on other components of the diet. Simple, cross-sectional analysis of dietary data from populations has shown an inverse relationship between the intake of free sugars and the intake of fat (91), suggesting that reducing free sugars might lead to an increase in fat intake. There is, however, a growing body of evidence from studies over time that shows that changes in intake of fat and free sugars are not inversely related, and that reductions in intake of fat are offset by increases in intakes of starch rather than free sugars (92, 93). Cole-Hamilton et al. (94) found that the intake of both fat and added sugars simultaneously decreased as fibre intake increased. Overall dietary goals that promote increased intake of wholegrain staple foods, fruits and vegetables and a reduced consumption of free sugars are thus unlikely to lead to an increased consumption of fat.

Influence of fluoride. Fluoride undoubtedly protects against dental caries (95). The inverse relationship between fluoride in drinking-water and dental caries, for instance, is well established. Fluoride reduces caries in children by between 20% and 40%, but does not eliminate dental caries altogether.

Over 800 controlled trials of the effect of fluoride administration on dental caries have been conducted; collectively these studies demonstrate that fluoride is the most effective preventive agent against caries (95). Several studies have that indicated that a relationship between sugars intake and caries still exists in the presence of adequate fluoride exposure (33, 71, 96, 97). In two major longitudinal studies in children, the observed relationships between sugars intake and development of dental caries remained even after controlling for use of fluoride and oral hygiene practices (66, 67). As mentioned earlier, following a review of available longitudinal studies, Marthaler (68) concluded that, even when preventive measures such as use of fluoride are employed, a relationship between sugars intake and caries still exists. He also stated that in industrialized countries where there is adequate exposure to fluoride, no further reduction in the prevalence and severity of dental caries will be achieved unless the intake of sugars is reduced.

A recent systematic review that investigated the importance of sugars intake in caries etiology in populations exposed to fluoride concluded that where there is adequate exposure to fluoride, sugars consumption is a moderate risk factor for caries in most people; moreover sugars consumption is likely to be a more powerful indicator for risk of caries in persons who do not have regular exposure to fluoride. Thus, restricting sugars consumption still has a role to play in the prevention of caries in situations where there is widespread use of fluoride but this role is not as strong as it is without exposure to fluoride (98). Despite the indisputable preventive role of fluoride, there is no strong evidence of a clear relationship between oral cleanliness and levels of dental caries (99–100).

Excess ingestion of fluoride during enamel formation can lead to dental fluorosis. This condition is observed particularly in countries that have high levels of fluoride in water supplies (95).

Starches and dental caries
Epidemiological studies have shown that starch is of low risk to dental caries. People who consume high-starch/low-sugars diets generally have low levels of caries, whereas people who consume low-starch/high-sugars diets have high levels of caries (39, 48, 49, 51, 67, 101, 102). In Norway and Japan the intake of starch increased during the Second World War, yet the occurrence of caries was reduced.

The heterogeneous nature of starch (i.e. degree of refinement, botanical origin, raw or cooked) is of particular relevance when assessing its potential cariogenicity. Several types of experiment have shown that raw starch is of low cariogenicity (103–105). Cooked starch is about one-third to one-half as cariogenic as sucrose (106, 107). Mixtures of starch and sucrose are, however, potentially more cariogenic than starch alone (108). Plaque pH studies, using an indwelling oral electrode, have shown starch-containing foods reduce plaque pH to below 5.5, but starches are less acidogenic than sucrose. Plaque pH studies measure acid production from a substrate rather than caries development, and take no account of the protective factors found in some starch-containing foods or of the effect of foods on stimulation of salivary flow.

Glucose polymers and pre-biotics are increasingly being added to foods in industrialized countries. Evidence on the cariogenicity of these carbohydrates is sparse and comes from animal studies, plaque pH studies and studies in vitro which suggest that maltodextrins and glucose syrups are cariogenic (109–111). Plaque pH studies and experiments in vitro suggest that isomalto-oligosaccharides and gluco-oligosaccharides may be less acidogenic than sucrose (*112–114*). There is, however, evidence that fructo-oligosaccharides are as acidogenic as sucrose (*115, 116*).

Fruit and dental caries

As habitually consumed, there is little evidence to show that fruit is an important factor in the development of dental caries (*67, 117–119*). A number of plaque pH studies have found fruit to be acidogenic, although less so than sucrose (*120–122*). Animal studies have shown that when fruit is consumed in very high frequencies (e.g. 17 times a day) it may induce caries (*123, 124*), but less so than sucrose. In the only epidemiological study in which an association between fruit consumption and DMFT was found (*125*), fruit intakes were very high (e.g. 8 apples or 3 bunches of grapes per day) and the higher DMFT in fruit farm workers compared with grain farm workers arose solely from differences in the numbers of missing teeth.

Dietary factors which protect against dental caries

Some dietary components protect against dental caries. The cariostatic nature of cheese has been demonstrated in several experimental studies (*126, 127*), and in human observational studies (*67*) and intervention studies (*128*). Cow's milk contains calcium, phosphorus and casein, all of which are thought to inhibit caries. Several studies have shown that the fall in plaque pH following milk consumption is negligible (*129, 130*). The cariostatic nature of milk has been demonstrated in animal studies (*131, 132*). Rugg-Gunn et al. (*67*) found an inverse relationship between the consumption of milk and caries increment in a study of adolescents in England. Wholegrain foods have protective properties; they require more mastication thereby stimulating increased saliva flow. Other foods that are good gustatory and/or mechanical stimulants to salivary flow include peanuts, hard cheeses and chewing gum. Both organic and inorganic phosphates (found in unrefined plant foods) have been found to be cariostatic in animal studies, but studies in humans have produced inconclusive results (*133, 134*). Both animal studies and experimental investigations in humans have shown that black tea extract increases plaque fluoride concentration and reduces the cariogenicity of a sugars-rich diet (*135, 136*).

Breastfeeding and dental caries

In line with the positive health effects of breastfeeding, epidemiological studies have associated breastfeeding with low levels of dental caries (*137, 138*). A few specific case studies have linked prolonged ad libitum and nocturnal breastfeeding to early childhood caries. Breastfeeding has the advantage that it does not necessitate the use of a feeder bottle, which has been associated with early childhood caries. A breastfed infant will also receive milk of a controlled composition to which additional free sugars have not been added. There are no benefits to dental health of feeding using a formula feed.

Dental erosion

Dental erosion is the progressive irreversible loss of dental hard tissue that is chemically etched away from the tooth surface by extrinsic and/or intrinsic acids by a process that does not involve bacteria. Extrinsic dietary acids include citric acid, phosphoric acid, ascorbic acid, malic acid, tartaric acid and carbonic acid found, for example, in fruits and fruit juices, soft drinks and vinegar. Erosion in severe cases leads to total tooth destruction (*139*). Human observational studies have shown an association between dental erosion and the consumption of a number of acidic foods and drinks, including frequent consumption of fruit juice, soft drinks (including sports drinks), pickles (containing vinegar), citrus fruits and berries (*140–144*). Age-related increases in dental erosion have been shown to be greater in those with the highest intake of soft drinks (*20*). Experimental clinical studies have shown that consumption of, or rinsing with, acidic beverages significantly lowers the pH of the oral fluids (*121*). Enamel is softened within one hour of exposure to cola but this may be reversed by exposure to milk or cheese (*145, 146*). Animal studies have shown that fruit and soft drinks cause erosion (*124, 147*), although fruit juices are significantly more destructive than whole fruits (*148, 149*).

5.6.4 *Strength of evidence*

The strength of the evidence linking dietary sugars to the risk of dental caries is in the multiplicity of the studies rather than the power of any individual study. Strong evidence is provided by the intervention studies (*50, 51*) but the weakness of these studies is that they were conducted in the pre-fluoride era. More recent studies also show an association between sugars intake and dental caries albeit not as strong as in the pre-fluoride era. However, in many developing countries people are not yet exposed to the benefits of fluoride.

Cross-sectional studies should be interpreted with caution because dental caries develop over time and therefore simultaneous measurements of disease levels and diet may not give a true reflection of the role of diet in the development of the disease. It is the diet several years earlier that may be responsible for current caries levels. Longitudinal studies (*66, 67*) that have monitored a change in caries experience and related this to dietary factors provide stronger evidence. Such studies have been conducted on populations with an overall high sugars intake but a low interindividual variation; this may account for the weak associations that have been reported.

The studies that overcome the problem of low variation in consumption of sugars are studies that have monitored dental caries following a marked change in diet, for example, those conducted on populations during the Second World War and studies of populations before and after the introduction of sugars into the diet. Such studies have shown clearly that changes in dental caries mirror changes in economic growth and increased consumption of free sugars. Sometimes changes in sugars consumption were accompanied by an increase in other refined carbohydrates. There are, however, examples where sugars consumption decreased and starch consumption increased yet levels of dental caries declined.

Strong evidence of the relationship between sugar availability and dental caries levels comes from worldwide ecological studies (26, 28). The limitations of these studies are that they use data on sugar availability and not actual intake, they do not measure frequency of sugars intake, and they assume that level of intake is equal throughout the population. Also, the values are for sucrose, yet many countries obtain a considerable amount of their total sugars from other sugars. These studies have only considered DMFT of 12-year-olds, not always from a representative sample of the population.

Caution needs to be applied when extrapolating the results of animal studies to humans because of differences in tooth morphology, plaque bacterial ecology, salivary flow and composition, and the form in which the diet is provided (usually powdered form in animal experiments). Nonetheless, animal studies have enabled the effect on caries of defined types, frequencies and amounts of carbohydrates to be studied.

Plaque pH studies measure plaque acid production, but the acidogenicity of a foodstuff cannot be taken as a direct measurement of its cariogenic potential. Plaque pH studies take no account of protective factors in foods, salivary flow and the effects of other components of the diet. Many of the plaque pH studies that show falls in pH below the critical value of 5.5 with fruits and cooked starchy foods have been conducted using the indwelling electrode technique. This electrode is recognized as being hypersensitive and non-discriminating, tending to give an "all or nothing" response to all carbohydrates (150).

Research has consistently shown that when annual sugar consumption exceeds 15 kg per person per year (or 40 g per person per day) dental caries increase with increasing sugar intake. When sugar consumption is below 10 kg per person per year (around 27 g per person per day), levels of dental caries are very low (26, 28, 29, 51, 151–158). Exposure to fluoride (i.e. where the proportion of fluoride in drinking-water is 0.7– 1.0 ppm, or where over 90% of toothpastes available contain fluoride) increases the safe level of sugars consumption.

Tables 14–17 summarize the evidence relating to diet, nutrition and dental diseases.

Table 14
Summary of strength of evidence linking diet to dental caries

Evidence	Decreased risk	No relationship	Increased risk
Convincing	Fluoride exposure (local and systematic)	Starch intake (cooked and raw starch foods, such as rice, potatoes and bread; excludes cakes, biscuits and snacks with added sugars)	Amount of free sugars Frequency of free sugars
Probable	Hard cheese Sugars-free chewing gum	Whole fresh fruit	
Possible	Xylitol Milk Dietary fibre		Undernutrition
Insufficient	Whole fresh fruit		Dried fruits

Table 15
Summary of strength of evidence linking diet to dental erosion

Evidence	Decreased risk	No relationship	Increased risk
Convincing			
Probable			Soft drinks and fruit juices
Possible	Hard cheese Fluoride		
Insufficient			Whole fresh fruit

Table 16
Summary of strength of evidence linking diet to enamel developmental defects

Evidence	Decreased risk	No relationship	Increased risk
Convincing	Vitamin D		Excess fluoride
Probable			Hypocalcaemia

Table 17
Summary of strength of evidence linking diet to periodontal disease

Evidence	Decreased risk	No relationship	Increased risk
Convincing	Good oral hygiene		Deficiency of vitamin C
Probable			
Possible			Undernutrition
Insufficient	Antioxidant nutrients	Vitamin E supplementation	Sucrose

5.6.5 *Disease-specific recommendations*

It is important to set a recommended maximum level for the consumption of free sugars; a low free sugars consumption by a population will translate into a low level of dental caries. Population goals enable the oral health risks of populations to be assessed and health promotion goals monitored.

The best available evidence indicates that the level of dental caries is low in countries where the consumption of free sugars is below 15–20 kg per person per year. This is equivalent to a daily intake of 40–55 g per person and the values equate to 6–10% of energy intake. It is of particular importance that countries which currently have low consumption of free sugars (< 15–20 kg per person per year) do not increase consumption levels. For countries with high consumption levels it is recommended that national health authorities and decision-makers formulate country-specific and community-specific goals for reduction in the amount of free sugars, aiming towards the recommended maximum of no more than 10% of energy intake.

In addition to population targets given in terms of the amount of free sugars, targets for the frequency of free sugars consumption are also important. The frequency of consumption of foods and/or drinks containing free sugars should be limited to a maximum of four times per day.

Many countries that are currently undergoing nutrition transition do not have adequate exposure to fluoride. There should be promotion of adequate fluoride exposure via appropriate vehicles, for example, affordable toothpaste, water, salt and milk. It is the responsibility of national health authorities to ensure implementation of feasible fluoride programmes for their country. Research into the outcome of alternative community fluoride programmes should be encouraged.

In order to minimize the occurrence of dental erosion, the amount and frequency of intake of soft drinks and juices should be limited. Elimination of undernutrition prevents enamel hypoplasia and the other potential effects of undernutrition on oral health (e.g. salivary gland atrophy, periodontal disease, oral infectious diseases).

References

1. Sheiham A. Dietary effects on dental diseases. *Public Health Nutrition,* 2001, 4:569–591.

2. Kelly M et al. *Adult dental health survey: oral health in the United Kingdom 1998.* London, The Stationery Office, 2000.

3. Chen M et al. *Comparing oral health systems: a second international collaborative study.* Geneva, World Health Organization, 1997.

4. Steele JG et al. *National Diet and Nutrition Survey: people aged 65 years and over. Vol. 2. Report of the oral health survey.* London, The Stationery Office, 1998.

5. Joshipura KJ, Willett WC, Douglass CW. The impact of edentulousness on food and nutrient intake. *Journal of the American Dental Association,* 1996, **127**:459–467.

6. Moynihan PJ et al. Intake of non-starch polysaccharide (dietary fibre) in edentulous and dentate persons: an observational study. *British Dental Journal,* 1994, **177**:243–247.

7. *Global Oral Health Data Bank.* Geneva, World Health Organization, 2001.

8. Fejerskov O, Baelum V. Changes in prevalence and incidence of the major oral diseases. In: Guggenheim B, Shapiro H, eds. *Oral biology at the turn of the century. Truth, misconcepts and challenges.* Zurich, Karger, 1998:1–9.

9. Pitts NB, Evans DJ. The dental caries experience of 5-year-old children in the United Kingdom. Surveys coordinated by the British Association for the Study of Community Dentistry in 1995/96. *Community Dental Health,* 1997, **14**:47–52.

10. Poulsen S. Dental caries in Danish children and adolescents 1988–94. *Community Dentistry and Oral Epidemiology,* 1996, **24**:282–285.

11. Frencken JE, Kalsbeek H, Verrips GH. Has the decline in dental caries been halted? Changes in caries prevalence amongst 6- and 12-year-old children in Friesland, 1973–1988. *International Dental Journal,* 1990, **40**:225–230.

12. Marthaler TM, O'Mullane DM, Vrbic V. The prevalence of dental caries in Europe 1990–1995. ORCA Saturday Afternoon Symposium 1995. *Caries Research,* 1996, **30**:237–255.

13. Leous P, Petersen PE. *Oral health status and oral health behaviour of children in Belarus.* Copenhagen, WHO Regional Office for Europe, 2000.

14. Szöke J, Petersen PE. Evidence of dental caries decline among children in an East European country (Hungary). *Community Dentistry and Oral Epidemiology,* 2000, **28**:155–160.

15. Petersen PE, Rusu M. *Oral health status of children in Romania, 2000.* Copenhagen, WHO Regional Office for Europe, 2001.

16. Kuzmina EM. *Oral health status of children and adults in the Russian Federation.* Moscow, Ministry of Health and WHO Collaborating Centre for Preventive Oral Care, 1999.

17. O'Mullane DM, ed. *Oral health systems in European Union Countries – Biomed project.* Cork, University of Cork, 1996.

18. Wang HY et al. The second national survey of oral health status of children and adults in China. *International Dental Journal,* 2002, **52**:283–290.

19. Petersen PE, Kaka M. Oral health status of children and adults in the Republic of Niger, Africa. *International Dental Journal,* 1999, **49**:159–164.

20. Walker A et al. *National Diet and Nutrition Survey: young people aged 4 to 18 years. Vol. 2. Report of the oral health survey.* London, The Stationery Office, 2000.

21. Rugg-Gunn AJ. *Nutrition and dental health.* Oxford, Oxford Medical Publications, 1993.

22. **Enwonwu CO.** Interface of malnutrition and periodontal diseases. *American Journal of Clinical Nutrition,* 1995, **61**(Suppl.):430–436.

23. **Enwonwu CO, Phillips RS, Falkler WA.** Nutrition and oral infectious diseases: state of the science. *Compendium of Continuing Education in Dentistry,* 2002, **23**:431–436.

24. **Arens U, ed.** *Oral health – diet and other factors: the Report of the British Nutrition Foundation's Task Force.* Amsterdam, Elsevier Science Publishing Company, 1999.

25. **Arends J, ten Bosch JJ.** In vivo de- and remineralisation of dental enamel. In: Leach SA, ed. *Factors relating to demineralisation and remineralisation of the teeth.* Oxford, IRL Press, 1986:1–11.

26. **Sreebny LM.** Sugar availability, sugar consumption and dental caries. *Community Dentistry and Oral Epidemiology,* 1982, **10**:1–7.

27. **Sreebny LM.** Sugar and human dental caries. *World Review of Nutrition and Dietetics,* 1982, **40**:19–65.

28. **Woodward M, Walker AR.** Sugar consumption and dental caries: evidence from 90 countries. *British Dental Journal,* 1994, **176**:297–302.

29. **Miyazaki H, Morimoto M.** Changes in caries prevalence in Japan. *European Journal of Oral Sciences,* 1996, **104**:452–458.

30. **Marthaler TM.** Epidemiological and clinical dental findings in relation to intake of carbohydrates. *Caries Research,* 1967, **1**:222–238.

31. **Takeuchi M.** Epidemiological study on dental caries in Japanese children before, during and after World War II. *International Dental Journal,* 1961, **11**:443–457.

32. **Sognnaes RF.** Analysis of wartime reduction of dental caries in European children. *American Journal of Diseases of Childhood,* 1948, **75**:792–821.

33. **Weaver R.** Fluorine and wartime diet. *British Dental Journal,* 1950, **88**:231–239.

34. **Bang G, Kristoffersen T.** Dental caries and diet in an Alaskan Eskimo population. *Scandinavian Journal of Dental Research,* 1972, **80**:440–444.

35. **Olsson B.** Dental health situation in privileged children in Addis Ababa, Ethiopia. *Community Dentistry and Oral Epidemiology,* 1979, **7**:37–41.

36. **MacGregor AB.** Increasing caries incidence and changing diet in Ghana. *International Dental Journal,* 1963, **13**:516–522.

37. **Sheiham A.** The prevalence of dental caries in Nigerian populations. *British Dental Journal,* 1967, **123**:144–148.

38. **Emslie RD.** A dental health survey in the Republic of the Sudan. *British Dental Journal,* 1966, **120**:167–178.

39. **Fisher FJ.** A field study of dental caries, periodontal disease and enamel defects in Tristan da Cunha. *British Dental Journal,* 1968, **125**:447–453.

40. **Roberts IF, Roberts GJ.** Relation between medicines sweetened with sucrose and dental disease. *British Medical Journal,* 1979, **2**:14–16.

41. **Masalin K, Murtamaa H, Meurman JH.** Oral health of workers in the modern Finnish confectionery industry. *Community Dentistry and Oral Epidemiology,* 1990, **18**:126–130.

42. Petersen PE. Dental health among workers at a Danish chocolate factory. *Community Dentistry and Oral Epidemiology*, 1983, 11:337–341.

43. Katayama T et al. Incidence and distribution of *Strep mutans* in plaque from confectionery workers. *Journal of Dental Research*, 1979, 58:2251.

44. Anaise JZ. Prevalence of dental caries among workers in the sweets industry in Israel. *Community Dentistry and Oral Epidemiology*, 1978, 6:286–289.

45. Bradford EW, Crabb HSM. Carbohydrates and the incidence of caries in the deciduous dentition. In: Hardwick JL, Dustin A, Held HR, eds. *Advances in fluoride research and dental caries prevention*. London, Pergamon, 1963:319–323.

46. Bradford EW, Crabb HSM. Carbohydrate restriction and caries incidence: a pilot study. *British Dental Journal*, 1961, 111:273–279.

47. Silverstein SJ et al. Dental caries prevalence in children with a diet free of refined sugar. *American Journal of Public Health*, 1983, 73:1196–1199.

48. Harris R. Biology of the children of Hopewood House, Bowral, Australia. IV. Observations on dental caries experience extending over 5 years (1957–61). *Journal of Dental Research*, 1963, 42:1387–1399.

49. Newbrun E et al. Comparison of dietary habits and dental health of subjects with hereditary fructose intolerance and control subjects. *Journal of the American Dental Association*, 1980, 101:619–626.

50. Gustafsson BE et al. The Vipeholm dental caries study. The effect of different levels of carbohydrate intake on caries activity in 436 individuals observed for 5 years. *Acta Odontologica Scandinavica*, 1954, 11:232–364.

51. Scheinin A, Makinen KK, Ylitalo K. Turku sugar studies. V. Final report on the effect of sucrose, fructose and xylitol diets on the caries incidence in man. *Acta Odontologica Scandinavica*, 1976, 34:179–198.

52. Garn SM et al. Relationships between sugar-foods and DMFT in 1968–1970. *Ecology of Food and Nutrition*, 1980, 9:135–138.

53. Granath LE et al. Variation in caries prevalence related to combinations of dietary and oral hygiene habits and chewing fluoride tablets in 4-year-old children. *Caries Research*, 1978, 12:83–92.

54. Schröder U, Granath LE. Dietary habits and oral hygiene as predictors of caries in 3-year-old children. *Community Dentistry and Oral Epidemiology*, 1983, 11:308–311.

55. Hausen H, Heinonen OP, Paunio I. Modification of occurrence of caries in children by toothbrushing and sugar exposure in fluoridated and non-fluoridated area. *Community Dentistry and Oral Epidemiology*, 1981, 9:103–107.

56. Peng B et al. Oral health status and oral health behaviour of 12-year-old urban schoolchildren in the People's Republic of China. *Community Dental Health*, 1997, 14:238–244.

57. Petersen PE. Oral health behaviour of 6-year-old Danish children. *Acta Odontologica Scandinavica*, 1992, 50:57–64.

58. Petersen PE, Razanamihaja N. Oral health status of children and adults in Madagascar. *International Dental Journal*, 1996, 46:41–47.

59. Petersen PE et al. Dental caries and dental health behaviour situation among 6- and 12-year-old urban schoolchildren in Madagascar. *African Dental Journal*, 1991, 5:1–7.

60. Al-Tamimi S, Petersen PE. Oral health situation of schoolchildren, mothers and schoolteachers in Saudi Arabia. *International Dental Journal,* 1998, 48:180–186.

61. Persson LA et al. Infant feeding and dental caries – a longitudinal study of Swedish children. *Swedish Dental Journal,* 1985, 9:201–206.

62. Stecksen-Blicks C, Holm AK. Dental caries, tooth trauma, malocclusion, fluoride usage, toothbrushing and dietary habits in 4-year-old Swedish children: changes between 1967 and 1992. *International Journal of Paediatric Dentistry,* 1995, 5:143–148.

63. Petersen PE et al. Oral health status and oral health behaviour of urban and rural schoolchildren in Southern Thailand. *International Dental Journal,* 2001, 51:95–102.

64. Hinds K, Gregory J. *National Diet and Nutrition Survey: children aged 1.5–4.5 years. Vol. 2. Report of the dental survey.* London, Her Majesty's Stationery Office, 1995.

65. Stecksen-Blicks C, Gustafsson L. Impact of oral hygiene and use of fluorides on caries increment in children during one year. *Community Dentistry and Oral Epidemiology,* 1986,14:185–189.

66. Burt BA et al. The effects of sugars intake and frequency of ingestion on dental caries increment in a three-year longitudinal study. *Journal of Dental Research,* 1988, 67:1422–1429.

67. Rugg-Gunn AJ et al. Relationship between dietary habits and caries increment assessed over two years in 405 English adolescent schoolchildren. *Archives of Oral Biology,* 1984, 29:983–992.

68. Marthaler T. Changes in the prevalence of dental caries: how much can be attributed to changes in diet? *Caries Research,* 1990, 24(Suppl.):3–15.

69. Rose G. *The strategy of preventive medicine.* Oxford, Oxford University Press, 1993.

70. Holbrook WP et al. Longitudinal study of caries, cariogenic bacteria and diet in children just before and after starting school. *European Journal of Oral Sciences,* 1995, 103:42–45.

71. Holt RD. Foods and drinks at four daily time intervals in a group of young children. *British Dental Journal,* 1991, 170:137–143.

72. Holbrook WP et al. Caries prevalence, *Streptococcus mutans* and sugar intake among 4-year-old urban children in Iceland. *Community Dentistry and Oral Epidemiology,* 1989, 17:292–295.

73. Firestone AR, Schmid R, Muhlemann HR. Effect of the length and number of intervals between meals on caries in rats. *Caries Research,* 1984, 18:128–133.

74. König KG, Schmid P, Schmid R. An apparatus for frequency-controlled feeding of small rodents and its use in dental caries experiments. *Archives of Oral Biology,* 1968, 13:13–26.

75. Karlsbeek H, Verrips GH. Consumption of sweet snacks and caries experience of primary school children. *Caries Research,* 1994, 28:477–483.

76. Sundin B, Granath L, Birkhed D. Variation of posterior approximal caries incidence with consumption of sweets with regard to other caries-related

factors in 15–18-year-olds. *Community Dentistry and Oral Epidemiology,* 1992, 20:76–80.

77. Bjarnason S, Finnbogason SY, Noren JG. Sugar consumption and caries experience in 12- and 13-year-old Icelandic children. *Acta Odontologica Scandinavica,* 1989, 47:315–321.

78. Hankin JH, Chung CS, Kau MC. Genetic and epidemiological studies of oral characteristics in Hawaii's school children: dietary patterns and caries prevalence. *Journal of Dental Research,* 1973, 52:1079–1086.

79. Hefti A, Schmid R. Effect on caries incidence in rats of increasing dietary sucrose levels. *Caries Research,* 1979, 13:298–300.

80. Mikx FH et al. Effect of *Actinomyces viscosus* on the establishment and symbiosis of *Streptococcus mutans* and *Streptococcus sanguis* on SPF rats on different sucrose diets. *Caries Research,* 1975, 9:1–20.

81. Guggenheim B et al. The cariogenicity of different dietary carbohydrates tested on rats in relative gnotobiosis with a *Streptococcus* producing extracellular polysaccharide. *Helvetica Odontologica Acta,* 1966, 10:101–113.

82. Gustafsson G et al. Experimental dental caries in golden hamsters. *Odontolgisk Tidskrift,* 1953, 61:386–399.

83. Szpunar SM, Eklund SA, Burt BA. Sugar consumption and caries risk in schoolchildren with low caries experience. *Community Dentistry and Oral Epidemiology,* 1995, 23:142–146.

84. Kleemola-Kujala E, Rasanen L. Relationship of oral hygiene and sugar consumption to risk of caries in children. *Community Dentistry and Oral Epidemiology,* 1982, 10:224–233.

85. Jamel HA et al. Sweet preference, consumption of sweet tea and dental caries: studies in urban and rural Iraqi populations. *International Dental Journal,* 1997, 47:213–217.

86. Rodrigues C, Watt RG, Sheiham A. The effects of dietary guidelines on sugar intake and dental caries in 3-year-olds attending nurseries. *Health Promotion International,* 1999, 14:329–335.

87. Cleaton-Jones P et al. Dental caries and sucrose intake in five South African pre-school groups. *Community Dentistry and Oral Epidemiology,* 1984, 12:381–385.

88. Ismail AI, Burt BA, Eklund SA. The cariogenicity of soft drinks in the United States. *Journal of the American Dental Association,* 1984, 109:241–245.

89. Jenkins GN, Ferguson DB. Milk and dental caries. *British Dental Journal,* 1966, 120:472–477.

90. Frostell G et al. Effect of partial substitution of invert sugar for sucrose in combination with Duraphat treatment on caries development in pre-school children: the Malmo Study. *Caries Research,* 1991, 25:304–310.

91. Gibney M et al. Consumption of sugars. *American Journal of Clinical Nutrition,* 1995, 62(Suppl.1):178–194 (erratum appears in *American Journal of Clinical Nutrition,* 1997, 65:1572–1574).

92. Alexy U, Sichert-Hellert W, Kersting M. Fifteen-year time trends in energy and macronutrient intake in German children and adolescents: results of the DONALD study. *British Journal of Nutrition,* 2002, 87:595–604.

93. Fletcher ES, Adamson AJ, Rugg-Gunn AJ. Twenty years of change in the dietary intake and BMI of Northumbrian adolescents. *Proceedings of the Nutrition Society,* 2001, **60**:171A–237A.

94. Cole-Hamilton I et al. A study among dietitians and adult members of their households of the practicalities and implications of following proposed dietary guidelines for the UK. British Dietetic Association Community Nutrition Group Nutrition Guidelines Project. *Human Nutrition – Applied Nutrition,* 1986, **40**:365–389.

95. *Fluorides and oral health. Report of a WHO Expert Committee on Oral Health Status and Fluoride Use.* Geneva, World Health Organization, 1994 (WHO Technical Report Series, No. 846).

96. Künzel W, Fischer T. Rise and fall of caries prevalence in German towns with different F concentrations in drinking water. *Caries Research,* 1997, **31**:166–173.

97. Beighton D, Adamson A, Rugg-Gunn A. Associations between dietary intake, dental caries experience and salivary bacterial levels in 12-year-old English schoolchildren. *Archives of Oral Biology,* 1996, **41**:271–280.

98. Burt BA, Pai S. Sugar consumption and caries risk: a systematic review. *Journal of Dental Education,* 2001, **65**: 1017–1023.

99. Sutcliffe P. Oral cleanliness and dental caries. In: Murray JJ, ed. *The prevention of oral disease.* Oxford, Oxford University Press, 1996:68–77.

100. Bellini HT, Arneberg P, von der Fehr FR. Oral hygiene and caries. A review. *Acta Odontologica Scandinavica,* 1981, **39**:257–265.

101. Russell AL et al. Dental surveys in relation to nutrition. *Public Health Reports,* 1960, **75**:717–723.

102. Afonsky D. Some observations on dental caries in central China. *Journal of Dental Research,* 1951, **30**:53–61.

103. Brudevold F et al. Intraoral demineralisation and maltose clearance from wheat starch. *Caries Research,* 1985, **19**:136–144.

104. Grenby TH. Effects of starch and sugar diets on dental caries. A comparison of two different methods of assessing caries in rodents. *British Dental Journal,* 1970, **128**:575–578.

105. Grenby TH. The effects of some carbohydrates on experimental dental caries in the rat. *Archives of Oral Biology,* 1963, **8**:27–30.

106. Bowen WH et al. A method to assess cariogenic potential of foodstuffs. *Journal of the American Dental Association,* 1980, **100**:677–681.

107. Koulourides T et al. Cariogenicity of nine sugars tested with an intraoral device in man. *Caries Research,* 1976, **10**:427–441.

108. Firestone AR, Schmid R, Muhlemann HR. Cariogenic effects of cooked wheat starch alone or with sucrose and frequency-controlled feeding in rats. *Archives of Oral Biology,* 1982, **27**:759–763.

109. Grenby TH, Mistry M. Properties of maltodextrins and glucose syrups in experiments in vitro and in the diets of laboratory animals, relating to dental health. *British Journal of Nutrition,* 2000, **84**:565–574.

110. Moynihan PJ et al. Effect of glucose polymers in water, milk and a milk substitute on plaque pH in vitro. *International Journal of Paediatric Dentistry,* 1996, **6**:19–24.

111. Grenby TH. The effect of glucose syrup on dental caries in the rat. *Caries Research*, 1972, 6:52–69.

112. Koga T et al. Effects of panose on glucan synthesis and cellular adherence by *Streptococcus mutans*. *Microbiology and Immunology*, 1988, 32:25–31.

113. Ooshima T et al. The caries inhibitory effect of GOS-sugar in vitro and rat experiments. *Microbiology and Immunology*, 1988, 32:1093–1105.

114. Roberts KR, Hayes ML. Effects of 2-deoxy-D-glucose and other sugar analogues on acid production from sugars by human dental plaque bacteria. *Scandinavian Journal of Dental Research*, 1980, 88:201–209.

115. Moynihan PJ et al. Acidogenic potential of fructo-oligosaccharides: incubation studies and plaque pH studies. *Caries Research*, 2001, 35:265–316.

116. Hartemink R et al. Degradation and fermentation of fructo-oligosaccharides by oral streptococci. *Journal of Applied Bacteriology*, 1995, 79:551–557.

117. Clancy KL et al. Snack food intake of adolescents and caries development. *Journal of Dental Research*, 1977, 56:568–573.

118. Martinsson T. Socio-economic investigation of school children with high and low caries frequency. 3. A dietary study based on information given by the children. *Odontologisk Revy*, 1972, 23:93–113.

119. Savara BS, Suher T. Dental caries in children one to six years of age as related to socio-economic level, food habits and toothbrushing. *Journal of Dental Research*, 1955, 34:870–875.

120. Hussein I, Pollard MA, Curzon ME. A comparison of the effects of some extrinsic and intrinsic sugars on dental plaque pH. *International Journal of Paediatric Dentistry*, 1996, 6:81–86.

121. Imfeld TN. *Identification of low caries risk dietary components*. Zurich, Karger, 1983 (Monographs in Oral Science, Vol. 11).

122. Ludwig TG, Bibby BG. Acid production from different carbohydrate foods in plaque and saliva. *Journal of Dental Research*, 1957, 36:56–60.

123. Imfeld T et al. Cariogenicity of Milchschnitte (Ferrero-GmbH) and apple in program-fed rats. *Caries Research*, 1991, 25:352–358.

124. Stephan RM. Effects of different types of human foods on dental health in experimental animals. *Journal of Dental Research*, 1966, 45:1551–1561.

125. Grobler SR, Blignaut JB. The effect of a high consumption of apples or grapes on dental caries and periodontal disease in humans. *Clinical Preventive Dentistry*, 1989,11:8–12.

126. Moynihan PJ, Ferrier S, Jenkins GN. The cariostatic potential of cheese: cooked cheese-containing meals increase plaque calcium concentration. *British Dental Journal*, 1999, 187:664–667.

127. Rugg-Gunn AJ et al. The effect of different meal patterns upon plaque pH in human subjects. *British Dental Journal*, 1975, 139:351–356.

128. Gedalia I et al. Dental caries protection with hard cheese consumption. *American Journal of Dentistry*, 1994, 7:331–332.

129. Rugg-Gunn AJ, Roberts GJ, Wright WG. Effect of human milk on plaque pH in situ and enamel dissolution in vitro compared with bovine milk, lactose and sucrose. *Caries Research*, 1985, 19:327–334.

130. Frostell G. Effects of milk, fruit juices and sweetened beverages on the pH of dental plaques. *Acta Odontologica Scandinavica,* 1970, **28**:609–622.

131. Bowen WH et al. Influence of milk, lactose-reduced milk, and lactose on caries in desalivated rats. *Caries Research,* 1991, **25**:283–286.

132. Reynolds EC, Johnson IH. Effect of milk on caries incidence and bacterial composition of dental plaque in the rat. *Archives of Oral Biology,* 1981, 26:445–451.

133. Nizel AE, Harris RS. The effects of phosphates on experimental dental caries: a literature review. *Journal of Dental Research,* **43**(Suppl. 6):1123–1136.

134. Craig GC. The use of a calcium sucrose phosphates–calcium orthophosphate complex as a cariostatic agent. *British Dental Journal,* 1975, **138**:25–28.

135. Lingstrom P, Wu CD, Wefel JS. In vivo effects of black tea infusion on dental plaque. *Journal of Dental Research,* 2000, **79**:594.

136. Linke HAB et al. Effect of black tea on caries formation in hamsters. *Journal of Dental Research,* 2000, **79**:594.

137. Silver DH. A longitudinal study of infant feeding practice, diet and caries, related to social class in children aged 3 and 8–10 years. *British Dental Journal,* 1987, **163**:296–300.

138. Holt RD, Joels D, Winter GB. Caries in pre-school children. The Camden study. *British Dental Journal,* 1982, **153**:107–109.

139. Meurman JH, ten Cate JM. Pathogenesis and modifying factors of dental erosion. *European Journal of Oral Sciences,* 1996, **104**:199–206.

140. Millward A et al. The distribution and severity of tooth wear and the relationship between erosion and dietary constituents in a group of children. *International Journal of Paediatric Dentistry,* 1994, **4**:151–157.

141. Järvinen VK, Rytomaa II, Heinonen OP. Risk factors in dental erosion. *Journal of Dental Research,* 1991, **70**:942–947.

142. Linkosalo E, Markkanen H. Dental erosions in relation to lactovegetarian diet. *Scandinavian Journal of Dental Research,* 1985, **93**:436–441.

143. Stabholz A et al. Tooth enamel dissolution from erosion or etching and subsequent caries development. *Journal of Pedodontics,* 1983, 7:100–108.

144. Thomas AE. Further observations on the influence of citrus fruit juices on human teeth. *New York State Dental Journal,* 1957, **23**:424–430.

145. Gedalia I et al. Enamel softening with Coca-Cola and rehardening with milk or saliva. *American Journal of Dentistry,* 1991, **4**:120–122.

146. Gedalia I et al. Tooth enamel softening with a cola type drink and rehardening with hard cheese or stimulated saliva in situ. *Journal of Oral Rehabilitation,* 1991, 18:501–506.

147. Holloway PJ, Mellanby M, Stewart RJC. Fruit drinks and tooth erosion. *British Dental Journal,* 1958, **104**:305–309.

148. Grenby TH, Mistry M, Desai T. Potential dental effects of infants fruit drinks studied in vitro. *British Journal of Nutrition,* 1990, **64**:273–283.

149. Miller CD. Erosion of molar teeth by acid beverages. *Journal of Nutrition,* 1950, 41:63–71.

150. Edgar WM. Prediction of the cariogenicity of various foods. *International Dental Journal,* 1985, **35**:190–194.

151. Ruxton CH, Garceau FJ, Cottrell RC. Guidelines for sugar consumption in Europe. Is a quantitative approach justified? *European Journal of Clinical Nutrition,* 1999, **53**:503–513.

152. Rodrigues CS. *Dietary guidelines, sugar intake and caries increment. A study in Brazilian nursery school children* [Thesis]. London, University of London, 1997.

153. Sheiham A. Sugars and dental decay. *Lancet,* 1983, **1**:282–284.

154. Buttner. Zuckeraufnahme und Karies. [Sugar intake and caries.] In: Cremer HD, ed. *Grundfragen der Ernährungswissenschaft. [Basics of nutrition.]* Freiburg im Breisgau, Rombach, 1971:175–191. [Cited by Marthaler TM. In: Guggenheim B, ed. *Health and sugar substitutes. Proceedings of the European Research Group for Oral Biology Conference on Sugar Substitutes, Geneva, Switzerland, 30 October – 1 November, 1978.* Basel, Karger, 1979:27–34.]

155. Takeuchi M. On the epidemiological principles in dental caries attack. *Bulletin of the Tokyo Dental College,* 1962, **3**:96–111.

156. Takahashi K. Statistical study on caries incidence in the first molar in relation to the amount of sugar consumption. *Bulletin of the Tokyo Dental College,* 1961, **2**:44–57.

157. Schulerud A. *Dental caries and nutrition during wartime in Norway.* Oslo, Fabritius og Snners Trykkeri, 1950.

158. Knowles EM. The effects of enemy occupation on the dental condition of children in the Channel Islands. *Monthly Bulletin of the Ministry of Health and the Public Health Laboratory Service,* 1946:161–172.

5.7 Recommendations for preventing osteoporosis

5.7.1 *Background*

Osteoporosis is a disease affecting many millions of people around the world. It is characterized by low bone mass and micro-architectural deterioration of bone tissue, leading to bone fragility and a consequent increase in risk of fracture (*1, 2*).

The incidence of vertebral and hip fractures increases exponentially with advancing age (while that of wrist fractures levels off after the age of 60 years) (*3*). Osteoporosis fractures are a major cause of morbidity and disability in older people and, in the case of hip fractures, can lead to premature death. Such fractures impose a considerable economic burden on health services worldwide (*4*).

5.7.2 *Trends*

Worldwide variation in the incidence and prevalence of osteoporosis is difficult to determine because of problems with definition and diagnosis. The most useful way of comparing osteoporosis prevalence between populations is to use fracture rates in older people. However, because osteoporosis is usually not life-threatening, quantitative data from developing countries are scarce. Despite this, the current consensus is that approximately 1.66 million hip fractures occur each year worldwide, that the incidence is set to increase four-fold by 2050 because of the increasing numbers of older people, and that the age-adjusted incidence rates are many times higher in affluent developed countries than in sub-Saharan Africa and Asia (*5–7*).

In countries with a high fracture incidence, rates are greater among women (by three- to four-fold). Thus, although widely regarded in these countries as a disease that affects women, 20% of symptomatic spine fractures and 30% of hip fractures occur in men (*8*). In countries where fracture rates are low, men and women are more equally affected (*7, 9–11*). The incidence of vertebral and hip fractures in both sexes increases exponentially with age. Hip-fracture rates are highest in Caucasian women living in temperate climates, are somewhat lower in women from Mediterranean and Asian countries, and are lowest in women in Africa (*9, 10, 12*). Countries in economic transition, such as Hong Kong Special Administrative Region (SAR) of China, have seen significant increases in age-adjusted fracture rates in recent decades, while the rates in industrialized countries appear to have reached a plateau (*13, 14*).

5.7.3 *Diet, physical activity and osteoporosis*

Diet appears to have only a moderate relationship to osteoporosis, but calcium and vitamin D are both important, at least in older populations.

Calcium is one of the main bone-forming minerals and an appropriate supply to bone is essential at all stages of life. In estimating calcium requirements, most committees have used either a factorial approach, where calculations of skeletal accretion and turnover rates are combined with typical values for calcium absorption and excretion, or a variety of methods based on experimentally-derived balance data (*15, 16*). There has been considerable debate about whether current recommended intakes are adequate to maximize peak bone mass and to minimize bone loss and fracture risk in later life, and the controversies continue (*2, 12, 15–17*).

Vitamin D is obtained either from the diet or by synthesis in the skin under the action of sunlight. Overt vitamin D deficiency causes rickets in children and osteomalacia in adults, conditions where the ratio of mineral to osteoid in bone is reduced. Poor vitamin D status in the elderly, at plasma levels of 25-hydroxyvitamin D above those associated with osteomalacia, has been linked to age-related bone loss and osteoporotic fracture, where the ratio of mineral to osteoid remains normal.

Many other nutrients and dietary factors may be important for long-term bone health and the prevention of osteoporosis. Among the essential nutrients, plausible hypotheses for involvement with skeletal health, based on biochemical and metabolic evidence, can be made for zinc, copper, manganese, boron, vitamin A, vitamin C, vitamin K, the B vitamins, potassium and sodium (*15*). Evidence from physiological and clinical studies is largely lacking, and the data are often difficult to interpret because of potential size-confounding or bone remodelling transient effects.

5.7.4 *Strength of evidence*

For older people, there is convincing evidence for a reduction in risk for osteoporosis with sufficient intake of vitamin D and calcium together, and for an increase in risk with high consumption of alcohol and low body weight. Evidence suggesting a probable relationship, again in older people, supports a role for calcium and vitamin D separately, but none with fluoride.

Strength of evidence with fracture as outcome

There is considerable geographical variation in the incidence of fractures, and cultural variation in the intakes of nutrients associated with osteoporosis and the clinical outcome of fracture. In Table 18, where the evidence on risk factors for osteoporosis is summarized, it is important to note that the level of certainty is given in relation to fracture as the outcome, rather than apparent bone mineral density as measured by dual-energy X-ray absorptiometry or other indirect methods. Since the Consultation addressed health in terms of burden of disease, fractures were considered the more relevant end-point.

Table 18
Summary of strength of evidence linking diet to osteoporotic fractures

Evidence	Decreased risk	No relationship	Increased risk
Convincing Older people[a]	Vitamin D Calcium Physical activity		High alcohol intake Low body weight
Probable Older people[a]		Fluoride[b]	
Possible	Fruits and vegetables[c] Moderate alcohol intake Soy products	Phosphorus	High sodium intake Low protein intake (in older people) High protein intake

[a] In populations with high fracture incidence only. Applies to men and women older than 50-60 years, with a low calcium intake and/or poor vitamin D status.
[b] At levels used to fluoridate water supplies. High fluoride intake causes fluorosis and may also alter bone matrix.
[c] Several components of fruits and vegetables are associated with a decreased risk at levels of intake within the normal range of consumption (e.g. alkalinity, vitamin K, phytoestrogens, potassium, magnesium, boron). Vitamin C deficiency (scurvy) results in osteopenic bone disease.

5.7.5 *Disease-specific recommendations*

In countries with a high fracture incidence, a minimum of 400–500 mg of calcium intake is required to prevent osteoporosis. When consumption of dairy products is limited, other sources of calcium include fish with edible bones, tortillas processed with lime, green vegetables high in calcium (e.g. broccoli, kale), legumes and by-products of legumes (e.g. tofu). The interaction between calcium intake and physical activity, sun exposure, and intake of other dietary components (e.g. vitamin D, vitamin K, sodium, protein) and protective phytonutrients (e.g. soy compounds), needs to be considered before recommending increased calcium intake in countries with low fracture incidence in order to be in line with recommendations for industrialized countries (*18*).

With regard to calcium intakes to prevent osteoporosis, the Consultation referred to the recommendations of the Joint FAO/WHO Expert Consultation on Vitamin and Mineral Requirements in Human Nutrition (*18*) which highlighted the calcium paradox. The paradox (that hip fracture rates are higher in developed countries where calcium intake is higher than in developing countries where calcium intake is lower) clearly calls for an explanation. To date, the accumulated data indicate that the adverse effect of protein, in particular animal (but not vegetable) protein, might outweigh the positive effect of calcium intake on calcium balance.

The report of the Joint FAO/WHO Expert Consultation on Vitamin and Mineral Requirements in Human Nutrition made it clear that the recommendations for calcium intakes were based on long-term (90 days) calcium balance data for adults derived from Australia, Canada, the European Union, the United Kingdom and the United States, and were not necessarily applicable to all countries worldwide. The report also acknowledged that strong evidence was emerging that the requirements for calcium might vary from culture to culture for dietary, genetic, lifestyle and geographical reasons. Therefore, two sets of allowances were recommended: one for countries with low consumption of animal protein, and another based on data from North America and Western Europes (*18*).

The following conclusions were reached:

- There is no case for global, population-based approaches. A case can be made for targeted approaches with respect to calcium and vitamin D in high-risk subgroups of populations, i.e. those with a high fracture incidence.
- In countries with high osteoporotic fracture incidence, a low calcium intake (i.e. below 400–500 mg per day) (*15*) among older men and women is associated with increased fracture risk.
- In countries with high fracture incidence, increases in dietary vitamin D and calcium in the older populations can decrease fracture risk. Therefore, an adequate vitamin D status should be ensured. If vitamin D is obtained predominantly from dietary sources, for example, when sunshine exposure is limited, an intake of 5–10 µg per day is recommended.
- Although firm evidence is lacking, prudent dietary and some lifestyle recommendations developed in respect of other chronic diseases may prove helpful in terms of reducing fracture risk. These include:
  - increase physical activity;
  - reduce sodium intake;
  - increase consumption of fruits and vegetables;
  - maintain a healthy body weight;
  - avoid smoking;
  - limit alcohol intake.
- Convincing evidence indicates that physical activity, particularly activity that maintains or increases muscle strength, coordination and balance as important determinants of propensity for falling, is beneficial in prevention of osteoporotic fractures. In addition, regular lifetime weight-bearing activities, especially in modes that include impacts on bones and are done in vigorous fashion, increase peak bone mass in youth and help to maintain bone mass in later life.

References

1. **Consensus Development Conference.** Diagnosis, prophylaxis, and treatment of osteoporosis. *American Journal of Medicine*, 1993, **94**:646–650.
2. **Prentice A.** Is nutrition important in osteoporosis? *Proceedings of the Nutrition Society*, 1997, **56**:357–367.

3. **Compston JE**. Osteoporosis. In: Campbell GA, Compston JE, Crisp AJ, eds. *The management of common metabolic bone disorders.* Cambridge, Cambridge University Press, 1993:29–62.

4. **Johnell O**. The socioeconomic burden of fractures: today and in the 21st century. *American Journal of Medicine*, 1997, **103**(Suppl. 2A):S20–S25.

5. **Royal College of Physicians**. Fractured neck of femur. Prevention and management. Summary and recommendations of a report of the Royal College of Physicians. *Journal of the Royal College of Physicians*, 1989, **23**:8–12.

6. **Cooper C, Campion G, Melton LJ**. Hip fractures in the elderly: a world-wide projection. *Osteoporosis International,* 1992, **2**:285–289.

7. **Melton LJ III**. Epidemiology of fractures. In: Riggs BL, Melton LJ III, eds. *Osteoporosis: etiology, diagnosis, and management*, 2nd ed. Philadelphia, Lippincott-Raven, 1995: 225–247.

8. **Eastell R et al**. Management of male osteoporosis: report of the UK Consensus Group. *Quarterly Journal of Medicine*, 1998, **91**:71–92.

9. **Yan L et al**. Epidemiological study of hip fracture in Shenyang, People's Republic of China. *Bone*, 1999, **24**:151–155.

10. **Elffors L et al**. The variable incidence of hip fracture in southern Europe: the MEDOS Study. *Osteoporosis International*, 1994, **4**:253–263.

11. **Maggi S et al**. Incidence of hip fracture in the elderly: a cross-national analysis. *Osteoporosis International*, 1991, **1**:232–241.

12. *Osteoporosis: clinical guidelines for prevention and treatment*. London, Royal College of Physicians, 1999.

13. **Kannus P et al**. Epidemiology of hip fractures. *Bone*, 1996, **18**(Suppl.1): 57S–63S.

14. **Lau EM, Cooper C**. The epidemiology of osteoporosis: the oriental perspective in a world context. *Clinical Orthopaedics and Related Research*, 1996, **323**:65–74.

15. **Department of Health**. *Nutrition and bone health: with particular reference to calcium and vitamin D. Report of the Subgroup on Bone Health, Working Group on the Nutritional Status of the Population of the Committee on Medical Aspects of Food and Nutrition Policy*. London, The Stationery Office, 1998 (Report on Health and Social Subjects, No. 49).

16. **Standing Committee on the Scientific Evaluation of Dietary Reference Intakes, Food and Nutrition Board, Institute of Medicine**. *Dietary reference intakes for calcium, phosphorus, magnesium, vitamin D, and fluoride*. Washington, DC, National Academy Press, 1997.

17. **NIH Consensus Development Panel on Optimal Calcium Intake**. Optimal calcium intake. NIH Consensus Conference. *Journal of the American Medical Association*, 1994, **272**:1942–1948.

18. *Vitamin and mineral requirements in human nutrition. Report of the Joint FAO/ WHO Expert Consultation*. Geneva, World Health Organization, (in press).

6. Strategic directions and recommendations for policy and research

6.1 Introduction

The principal goal of public health policy is to give people the best chance to enjoy many years of healthy and active life. Public health action to prevent the adverse consequences of inappropriate dietary patterns and physical inactivity is now urgently needed. To this end, the Consultation discussed how nutrient/food intake and physical activity goals could be used by policy-makers to increase the proportion of people who make healthier choices about food and undertake sufficient physical activity to maintain appropriate body weights and adequate health status. This chapter discusses ways to catalyse the long-term changes that are needed to place people in a better position to make healthy choices about diet and physical activity. Such processes require long-term changes in thinking and action at the individual and societal levels; demand concerted action by national governments, international bodies, civil society and private entities and will need insights and energies contributed by multiple sectors of society.

New scientific information will be essential to permit adjustment not only of the policy levers, but also of the strategic processes to introduce change. This constitutes an important focus for applied research that should yield useful evidence to guide effective interventions.

Three key elements need to be analysed. The first is the range of possible policy principles that would help people achieve and maintain healthy dietary and activity patterns in a simple and rewarding manner. The second is the prerequisites for possible strategies to introduce these policies in different settings. These include the need for leadership, effective communication of problems and possible solutions, functioning alliances, and ways of encouraging enabling environments to facilitate change. The third is the possible strategic actions to promote healthy diets and physical activity.

6.2 Policy principles for the promotion of healthy diets and physical activity[1,2]

The Consultation recommended the consideration of the following policy principles when developing national strategies to reduce the burden of chronic diseases that are related to diet and physical inactivity.

- Strategies should be *comprehensive* and address all major dietary and physical activity risks for chronic diseases together, alongside other risks — such as tobacco use — from a multisectoral perspective.

- Each country should select what will constitute the *optimal mix of actions* that are in accord with national capabilities, laws and economic realities.

- *Governments have a central steering role* in developing strategies, ensuring that actions are implemented and monitoring their impact over the long term.

- *Ministries of health have a crucial convening role* — bringing together other ministries needed for effective policy design and implementation.

- *Governments need to work together with* the private sector, health professional bodies, consumer groups, academics, the research community and other nongovernmental bodies if sustained progress is to occur.

- *A life-course perspective* on chronic disease prevention and control is critical. This starts with maternal and child health, nutrition and care practices, and carries through to school and workplace environments, access to preventive health and primary care, as well as community-based care for the elderly and disabled people.

- Strategies should explicitly address equality and diminish disparities; they should focus on the needs of the *poorest communities and population groups* — this requires a strong role for government. Furthermore, since women generally make decisions about household nutrition, strategies should be *gender* sensitive.

---

[1] During the preparation of this report, by resolution WHA55.23 (*1*) in May 2002, the World Health Assembly called upon the Director-General to develop a global strategy on diet, physical activity and health (WHA55.23). The process for developing the WHO global strategy will involve formal consultation with Member States, United Nations agencies, civil society, and the private sector over a period of a year, prior to drafting a proposed global strategy for presentation to the Fifty-seventh World Health Assembly in 2004.

[2] Ensuring that people have access to adequate food which is safe and at the same time of appropriate nutritional quality is important. One of the commitments adopted by the *World Food Summit* convened by FAO in 1996, and reiterated in 2002 at the *World Food Summit: Five Years Later,* specifically endorses the implementation of policies aimed at "improving access by all, at all times to sufficient, nutritionally adequate and safe food".

- There are limits to what individual countries can do alone to promote optimal diets and healthy living. Strategies need to draw substantially on existing *international standards* that provide a reference in international trade. Member States may wish to see additional standards that address, for example, the marketing of unhealthy food (particularly those high in energy, saturated fat, salt and free sugars, and poor in essential nutrients) to children across national boundaries. Countries may also wish to consider means of ensuring the accessibility of healthier choices (such as fruits and vegetables) to all socioeconomic groups. WHO's international leadership role in pushing forward the agenda on diet, physical activity and health is crucial. FAO also has an important role in this process since it deals with issues relating to the production, trade, marketing of food and agricultural commodities and provides guidelines ensuring the safety and nutritional adequacy of food and food products.

6.3 Prerequisites for effective strategies

Drawing on experience with the implementation of local and national strategies for public health matters in different settings, the Expert Consultation concluded that there are a number of prerequisites for success. These include leadership, effective communication, functioning alliances and an enabling environment.

6.3.1 *Leadership for effective action*

Leadership is essential for introducing long-term changes. Within nations, governments have the primary responsibility for providing this leadership. In some cases leadership may be initiated by civil society organizations prior to government action. It is unlikely that there will be just one correct path to improved health: each country will need to determine the optimal mix of policies that its particular circumstances best fit. Each country will need to select measures within the reality of its economic and social resources. Within a given country, effective action may call for regional strategies.

More proactive leadership is needed, worldwide, to portray a holistic vision of food and nutritional issues as they affect overall health. Where this leadership has existed, it has been possible to make governments take notice and introduce the necessary changes. The question remains of how to develop and strengthen leadership capacity to reach a critical mass. The WHO collaborating centres in nutrition and the FAO network of centres of excellence are possible routes, although there is a clear need to strengthen existing capabilities.

Governments throughout the world have developed strategies to eradicate malnutrition, a term traditionally used synonymously with undernutrition. However, the growing problems of nutritional imbalance, overweight and obesity, together with their implications for the development of diabetes, cardiovascular problems and other diet-related noncommunicable diseases, are now at least as pressing. This applies especially to developing countries undergoing the nutrition transition; such countries bear a double burden of both overnutrition, as well as undernutrition and infectious diseases. Unless there is political commitment to spur governments on to achieve results, strategies cannot succeed. Setting population goals for nutrient intake and physical activity is necessary but insufficient. Giving people the best chance to enjoy many years of healthy and active life requires action at the community, family and individual levels.

6.3.2 *Effective communication*

Change can only be initiated through effective communication. The core role of health communication is to bridge the gap between technical experts, policy-makers and the general public. The proof of effective communications is its capacity to create awareness, improve knowledge and induce long-term changes in individual and social behaviours — in this case consumption of healthy diets and incorporating physical activity for health.

An effective health communication plan seeks to act on the opportunities at all stages of policy formulation and implementation, in order to positively influence public health. Sustained and well targeted communication will enable consumers to be better informed and make healthier choices. Informed consumers are better able to influence policy-makers; this was learned from work to limit the damage to health from tobacco use. Consumers can serve as advocates or may go on to lobby and influence their societies to bring about changes in supply and access to goods and services that support physical activity and nutritional goals.

The cost to the world of the current and projected epidemic of chronic disease related to diet and physical inactivity dwarfs all other health costs. If society can be mobilized to recognize those costs, policy-makers will eventually start confronting the issue and themselves become advocates of change. Experience shows that politicians can also be influenced by the positions taken by the United Nations agencies, and the messages that they promote. Medical networks have also been found to be effective advocates of change in the presence of a government that is responsive to the health needs of society. Consumer nongovernmental organizations and a wide variety of civil society organizations will also be critical in raising consumer consciousness and supporting the climate for constructive collaboration with the food industry and the private sector.

6.3.3 *Functioning alliances and partnerships*

Change can be accelerated if all groups in favour establish alliances to reach the common objective. Ideally, the effort should include a range of different parties whose actions influence people's options and choices about diet and physical activity. Alliances for action are likely to extend from communities to national and regional levels, involving formal focal points for nutrition within different public, private and voluntary bodies. The involvement of consumers associations is also important to facilitate health and nutrition education. International organizations with nutrition-related mandates, such as FAO and WHO, are expected to encourage the routing of reliable information through these networks. Alliances with other members of the United Nations family are also important — for example, with the United Nations Children's Fund on maternal — child nutrition and life-course approaches to health. Private sector industry with interests in food production, packaging, logistics, retailing and marketing, and other private entities concerned with lifestyles, sports, tourism, recreation, and health and life insurance, have a key role to play. Sometimes it is best to work with groups of industries rather than with individual industries that may wish to capitalize on change for their own benefit. All should be invited; those who share the health promotion objective will usually opt to participate in joint activities.

6.3.4 *Enabling environments*

Individual change is more likely to be facilitated and sustained if the macroenvironment and microenvironment within which choices are made support options perceived to be both healthy and rewarding. Food systems, marketing patterns and personal lifestyles should evolve in ways that make it easier for people to live healthier lives, and to choose the kinds of food that bring them the greatest health benefits. An enabling environment encompasses a wide frame of reference, from the environment at school, in the workplace and in the community, to transport policies, urban design policies, and the availability of a healthy diet. Furthermore, it requires supportive legislative, regulatory and fiscal policies to be in place. Unless there is an enabling context, the potential for change will be minimal. The ideal is an environment that not only promotes but also supports and protects healthy living, making it possible, for example, to bicycle or walk to work or school, to buy fresh fruits and vegetables, and eat and work in smoke-free rooms.

Specific actions to create enabling environments are outlined in greater detail below.

Supporting the availability and selection of nutrient-dense foods (fruits, vegetables, legumes, whole grains, lean meats and low-fat dairy products)
Within this overall concept, the issue of nutrient-dense foods versus energy-dense/nutrient-poor foods is critical as it concerns the balance between providing essential nourishment and maintaining a healthy weight. The quality of the fat and carbohydrate supplied also plays a key role. The following are all important: increasing access — especially of low-income communities — to a supply of nutrient-dense fresh foods; regulations that support this; facilitating access to high-quality diets through food pricing policies; nutrition labels to inform consumers, in particular about the appropriate use of health/nutrition claims. The provision of safe and nutritious food is now recognized not only as a human need but also as a basic right.

Assessing trends in changing consumption patterns and their implications for the food (agriculture, livestock, fisheries and horticulture) economy
Recommendations, which result in changes in dietary patterns, will have implications for all components of the food economy. Hence it is appropriate to examine trends in consumption patterns worldwide and deliberate on the potential of the food and agriculture sector to meet the demands and challenges posed by this report. All sectors in the food chain, from farm to the table, will have to be involved if the food economy is to respond to the need for changes in diets that will be necessary to cope with the burgeoning epidemic of noncommunicable diseases.

Hitherto most of the information on food consumption has been obtained from national Food Balance data. In order to understand better the relationship between food consumption patterns, diets and the emergence of noncommunicable diseases, it is crucial to obtain more reliable information on actual food consumption patterns and changing trends based on representative consumption surveys.

There is a need to monitor whether the guidelines developed in this report, and strategies based on them, will influence the behaviour of consumers and to what extent consumers will change their diets (and lifestyles) towards more healthy patterns.

The next step will be to assess the implications that these guidelines will have for agriculture, livestock, fisheries and horticulture. To meet the specified levels and patterns of consumption, new strategies may need to be developed. This assessment will need to include all stages in the food chain — from production and processing to marketing and consumption. The effects that these changes in the food economy could have on the sustainability of natural resource use would also need to be taken into account.

Likewise, international trade issues would need to be considered in the context of improving diets. Trade has an important role to play in improving food and nutrition security. Factors to consider include the impact of lower trade barriers on the purchasing power of consumers and variety of products available, while on the export side, questions of market access, competitiveness and income opportunities for domestic farmers and processors would merit attention. The impact that agricultural policy, particularly subsidies, has on the structure of production, processing and marketing systems and, ultimately, on the availability of foods that support healthy food consumption patterns will need to be examined.

Finally, assessments of the above issues, and more, will certainly have policy implications at both the national and international levels. These implications would need to be taken up in the appropriate forum and considered by the stakeholders concerned.

Sustainable development
The rapid increase in the consumption of animal-based foods, many of which are produced by intensive methods is likely to have a number of profound consequences. On the health side, increased consumption of animal products has led to higher intakes of saturated fats, which in conjunction with tobacco use, threatens to undermine the health gains made by reducing infectious diseases, in particular in the countries undergoing rapid economic and nutrition transition. Intensive cattle production also threatens the world's ability to feed its poorest people, who typically have very limited access to even basic foods. Environmental concerns abound too; intensive methods of animal rearing exert greater environmental pressures than traditional animal husbandry, largely because of the low efficiency in feed conversion and high water needs of cattle.

Intensive methods of livestock production may well provide much needed income opportunities, but this is often at the expense of the farmers' capacity to produce their own food. In contrast, the production of more diverse foods, in particular fruits, vegetables and legumes, may have a dual benefit in not only improving access to healthy foods but also in providing an alternative source of income for the farmer. This is further promoted if farmers can market their products directly to consumers, and thereby receive a greater proportion of final price. This model of food production can yield potent health benefits to both producers and consumers, and simultaneously reduce environmental pressures on water and land resources.

Agricultural policies in several countries often respond primarily to short-term commercial farming concerns rather than be guided by health and environmental considerations. For example, farm subsidies for beef and dairy production had good justification in the past — they provided improved access to high quality proteins but today contribute to human consumption patterns that may aggravate the burden of nutrition related chronic disease. This apparent disregard for the health consequences and environmental sustainability of present agricultural production, limits the potential for change in agricultural policies and food production, and at some point may lead to a conflict between meeting population nutrient intake goals and sustaining the demand for beef associated with the existing patterns of consumption. For example, if we project the consumption of beef in industrialized countries to the population of developing countries, the supply of grains for human consumption may be limited, specially for low-income groups.

Changes in agricultural policies which give producers an opportunity to adapt to new demands, increase awareness and empower communites to better address health and environmental consequences of present consumption patterns will be needed in the future. Integrated strategies aimed at increasing the responsiveness of governments to health and environmental concerns of the community will also be required. The question of how the world's food supply can be managed so as to sustain the demands made by population-size adjustments in diet is a topic for continued dialogue by multiple stake-holders that has major consequences for agricultural and environmental policies, as well as for world food trade.

Physical activity
A large proportion of the world's population currently takes an inadequate amount of physical activity to sustain physical and mental health. The heavy reliance on the motor car and other forms of labour-saving machinery has had much to do with this. Cities throughout the world have dedicated space for motor cars but little space for recreation. Changes in the nature of employment have meant that more time is spent travelling to and from work, thereby limiting the time available for the purchase and preparation of food. Cars are also contributors to growing urban problems, such as traffic congestion and air pollution.

Urban and workplace planners need to be more aware of the potential consequences of the progressive decline in occupational energy expenditure, and should be encouraged to develop transport and recreation policies that promote, support and protect physical activity. For example, urban planning, transportation and building design should give priority to the safety and transit of pedestrians and safe bicycle use.

Traditional diets

Modern marketing practices commonly displace local or ethnic dietary patterns. Global marketing, in particular, has wide-ranging effects on both consumer appetite for goods and perceptions of their value. While some traditional diets could benefit from thoughtful modification, research has shown that many are protective of health, and clearly environmentally sustainable. Much can be learned from these.

6.4 Strategic actions for promoting healthy diets and physical activity

The strategies for promoting healthy diets and physical activity need to reflect local and national realities as well as global determinants of diet and physical activity. They must be based on scientific evidence on the ways in which people's dietary and physical activity patterns have positive or adverse effects on health. In practice, strategies are likely to include at least some of the following practical actions.

6.4.1 *Surveillance of people's diets, physical activity and related disease burden*

A surveillance system for monitoring diet, physical activity and related health problems is essential to enable all interested stakeholders to track progress towards each country's diet-related health targets, and to guide the choice, intensity and timing of measures to accelerate achievement. The data required for implementing effective policies need to be specific for age, sex and social group, and indicate changing trends over time.

6.4.2 *Enabling people to make informed choices and take effective action*

Information about fat quality, salt and sugars content, and energy density should be incorporated into nutrition and health promotion messages, and as required in food labelling tailored to different population groups — including disadvantaged population groups — through the wide reach of modern media. The ultimate goal of information and communication strategies is to assure availability and choice of better quality food, access to physical activity and a better-informed global community.

6.4.3 *Making the best use of standards and legislation*

The Codex Alimentarius — the intergovernmental standard-setting body through which nations agree on standards for food — is currently being reviewed. Its work in the area of nutrition and labelling could be further strengthened to cover diet-related aspects of health. The feasibility of codes of practice in food advertising should also be explored.

6.4.4 *Ensuring that "healthy diet" components are available to all*

As consumers increase their preference for healthy diets, producers and suppliers will wish to orient their products and marketing to respond to this emerging demand. Governments could make it easier for consumers to exercise healthier choices, in accordance with the population nutrient intake goals given in this report by, for example, promoting the wider availability of food which is less processed and low in trans fatty acids, encouraging the use of vegetable oil for domestic consumers, and ensuring an adequate and sustainable supply of fish, fruits, vegetables and nuts in domestic markets.

In the case of meals prepared outside the home (i.e. in restaurants and fast-food outlets), information about their nutritional quality should be made available to consumers in a simple manner so that they can select healthier choices. For example, consumers should be able to ascertain not only the amount of fat or oil in the meals they have chosen, but also whether they are high in saturated fat or trans fatty acids.

6.4.5 *Achieving success through intersectoral initiatives*

Approaches to promoting healthy diets call for comprehensive strategies that cut across many sectors and involve the different groups within countries concerned with food, nutrition, agriculture, education, transport and other relevant policies. They should involve alliances that encourage the effective implementation of national and local strategies for healthy diets and physical activity. Intersectoral initiatives should encourage the adequate production and domestic supply of fruits, vegetables and wholegrain cereals, at affordable prices to all segments of the population, opportunities for all to access them regularly, and individuals to undertake appropriate levels of physical activity.

6.4.6 *Making the best of health services and the professionals who provide them*

The training of all health professionals (including physicians, nurses, dentists and nutritionists) should include diet, nutrition and physical activity as key determinants of medical and dental health. The social, economic, cultural and psychological determinants of dietary and physical activity choice should be included as integral elements of public health action. There is an urgent need to develop and strengthen existing training programmes to implement these actions successfully.

6.5 Call to action

There is now a large, convincing body of evidence that dietary patterns and the level of physical activity can not only influence existing health levels, but also determine whether an individual will develop chronic diseases such as cancer, cardiovascular disease and diabetes. These chronic diseases remain the main causes of premature death and disability in industrialized countries and in most developing countries. Developing countries are demonstrably increasingly at risk, as are the poorer populations of industrialized countries.

In communities, districts and countries where widespread, integrated interventions have been implemented, dramatic decreases in risk factors have occurred. Successes have come about where the public has acknowledged that the unnecessary premature deaths that occur in their community are largely preventable and have empowered themselves and their civic representatives to create health-supporting environments. This has been achieved most successfully by establishing a working relationship between communities and governments; through enabling legislation and local initiatives affecting schools and the workplace; by involving consumers' associations; and by involving food producers and the food-processing industry.

There is a need for data on current and changing trends in food consumption in developing countries, including research on what influences people's eating behaviour and physical activity and what can be done to address this. There is also a need, on a continuing basis, to develop strategies to change people's behaviour towards adopting healthy diets and lifestyles, including research on the supply and demand side related to this changing consumer behaviour.

Beyond the rhetoric, this epidemic can be halted — the demand for action must come from those affected. The solution is in our hands.

Reference

1. Resolution WHA55.23. Diet, physical activity and health. In: *Fifty-fifth World Health Assembly, Geneva, 13–18 May 2002. Volume 1. Resolutions and decisions, annexes*. Geneva, World Health Organization, 2002 (document WHA55/2002/REC/1):28–30.

Acknowledgements

Special acknowledgement was made by the Consultation to the following individuals who were instrumental in the preparation and proceedings of the meeting: Dr C. Nishida, Department of Nutrition for Health and Development, WHO, Geneva, Switzerland; Dr P. Puska, Director, Department of Noncommunicable Disease Prevention and Health Promotion, WHO, Geneva, Switzerland; Dr P. Shetty, Chief, Food and Nutrition Division, Rome, Italy; and Dr R. Weisel, Food and Nutrition Division, FAO, Rome, Italy.

The Consultation also expressed deep appreciation to the following individuals for their contributions to the running of the meeting and the finalizing of the report: Dr M. Deurenberg-Yap, Health Promotion Board, Singapore, Professor S. Kumanyika, University of Pennsylvania, Philadelphia, PA, USA; Professor J. C. Seidell, Free University of Amsterdam, Amsterdam, the Netherlands; and Dr R. Uauy, London School of Hygiene and Tropical Medicine, London, England and Institute of Nutrition of the University of Chile, Santiago, Chile.

The Consultation also thanked the authors of the background papers for the Consultation: Dr N. Allen, University of Oxford, Oxford, England; Dr P. Bennett, National Institute of Diabetes and Digestive and Kidney Diseases, Phoenix, AZ, USA; Professor I. Caterson, University of Sydney, Sydney, Australia; Dr I. Darnton-Hill, Columbia University, New York, NY, USA; Professor W.P.T. James, International Obesity Task Force, London, England; Professor M.B. Katan, Wageningen University, Wageningen, Netherlands; Dr T.J. Key, University of Oxford, Oxford, England; Dr J. Lindströmn, National Public Health Institute, Helsinki, Finland; Dr A. Louheranta, National Public Health Institute, Helsinki, Finland; Professor J. Mann, University of Otago, Dunedin, New Zealand; Dr P. Moynihan, University of Newcastle, Newcastle-upon-Tyne, England; Dr P.E. Petersen, Noncommunicable Disease and Health Promotion, WHO, Geneva, Switzerland; Dr A. Prentice, Medical Research Council Human Nutrition Research, Cambridge, England; Professor K.S. Reddy, All India Institute of Medical Science, New Delhi, India; Dr A. Schatzkin, National Institutes of Health, Bethesda, MD, USA; Dr A.P. Simopoulos, The Centre for Genetics, Nutrition and Health, Washington, DC, USA; Ms E. Spencer, University of Oxford, Oxford, England; Dr N. Steyn, Medical Research Council, Tygerberg, South Africa; Professor B. Swinburn, Deakin University, Melbourne, Victoria, Australia; Professor N. Temple, Athabasca University, Athabasca, Alberta, Canada; Ms R.Travis, University of Oxford, Oxford, England; Dr J.Tuomilehto, National Public Health Institute, Helsinki, Finland; Dr W. Willett, Harvard School of Public Health, Boston, MA, USA; and Professor P. Zimmet, International Diabetes Institute, Caulfield, Victoria, Australia.

The Consultation also recognized the valuable contributions made by the following individuals who provided comments on the background documents: Dr Franca Bianchini, Unit of Chemoprevention, International Agency for Research on Cancer, Lyon, France; Mr G. Boedeker, Economic and Social Department, FAO, Rome, Italy; Professor G.A. Bray, Pennington Biomedical Research Center, Louisiana State University, Baton Rouge, LA, USA; Mr J. Bruinsma, Economic and Social Department, FAO, Rome, Italy; Dr L.K. Cohen, National Institutes of Health, Bethesda, MD, USA; Professor A. Ferro-Luzzi, National Institute for Food and Nutrition Research, Rome, Italy; Dr R. Francis, Freeman Hospital, Newcastle-upon-Tyne, England; Dr Ghafoor-unissa, Indian Council of Medical Research, New Delhi, India; Dr K. Hardwick, National Institutes of Health, Bethesda, MD, USA; Dr H. King, Department of Management of Noncommunicable Diseases, WHO, Geneva, Switzerland; Dr J. King, University of California, Davis, CA, USA; Dr L.N. Kolonel, University of Hawaii, Manoa, HI, USA; Professor N.S. Levitt, University of Cape Town, Cape Town, South Africa; Dr P. Lingström, University of Gothenburg, Gothenburg, Sweden; Professor A. McMichael, Australian National University, Canberra, Australian Capital Territory, Australia; Professor S. Moss, Oral Health Promotion Committee, New York, NY, USA; Professor K. O'Dea, Menzies School of Health Research, Alice Springs, Northern Territory, Australia; Professor D. O'Mullane, University of Cork, Cork, Ireland; Dr P. Pietinen, National Public Health Institute, Helsinki, Finland; Dr J. Powles, University of Cambridge, Cambridge, England; Dr E. Riboli, International Agency for Research on Cancer, Lyon, France; Dr S. Rösnner, Huddinge University Hospital,

Huddinge, Sweden; Professor A. Rugg-Gunn, University of Newcastle, Newcastle-upon-Tyne, England; Mr J. Schmidhuber, Economic and Social Department, FAO, Rome, Italy; Professor A. Sheiham, University College London Medical School, London, England; Professor S. Truswell, University of Sydney, Sydney, New South Wales, Australia; Dr S. Tsugane, National Cancer Center Research Institute East, Tsukiji, Tokyo, Japan; Dr Ilkka Vuori, UKK Institute for Health Promotion Research, Tampere, Finland; Dr A.R.P. Walker, South African Institute for Medical Research, Johannesburg, South Africa; Dr S. Watanabe, Tokyo University of Agriculture, Tokyo, Japan; Dr C. Yajnik, King Edward Memorial Hospital Research Centre, Mumbai, India; and Dr S. Yusaf, McMaster University, Hamilton, Ontario, Canada.

Acknowledgement was made by the Consultation to the following individuals for their continual guidance: Dr D. Yach, Executive Director, Noncommunicable Diseases and Mental Health, WHO, Geneva, Switzerland; Dr D. Nabarro, Executive Director, Sustainable Development and Healthy Environments, WHO, Geneva, Switzerland; Mr H. De Haen, Assistant Director-General, Economic and Social Department, FAO, Rome, Italy; Dr G.A. Clugston, Director, Department of Nutrition for Health and Development, WHO, Geneva, Switzerland; and Dr K. Tontisirin, Director, Food and Nutrition Division, FAO, Rome, Italy.

The Consultation expressed special appreciation to Ms P. Robertson for her valuable contribution to the preparation and running of the meeting, to Mrs A. Haden and Mrs A. Rowe for their editorial assistance, and to Mrs R. Imperial Laue, Ms S. Nalty, Ms T. Mutru, Mrs R. Bourne, Mrs A. Manus, Mrs A. Ryan-Röhrich and Ms C. Melin for their assistance in checking, typing and finalizing the manuscript.

Annex

Summary of the strength of evidence for obesity, type 2 diabetes, cardiovascular disease (CVD), cancer, dental disease and osteoporosis[a]

	Obesity	Type 2 diabetes	CVD	Cancer	Dental disease	Osteoporosis
Energy and fats						
High intake of energy-dense foods	C↑					
Saturated fatty acids		P↑	C↑[b]			
Trans fatty acids			C↑			
Dietary cholesterol			P↑			
Myristic and palmitic acid			C↑			
Linoleic acid			C↓			
Fish and fish oils (EPA and DHA)			C↓			
Plant sterols and stanols			P↓			
α-Linolenic acid			P↓			
Oleic acid			P↓			
Stearic acid			P-NR			
Nuts (unsalted)			P↓			
Carbohydrate						
High intake of NSP (dietary fibre)	C↓	P↓	P↓			
Free sugars (frequency and amount)					C↑[c]	
Sugar-free chewing gum					P↓[c]	
Starch[d]					C-NR	
Wholegrain cereals			P↓			
Vitamins						
Vitamin C deficiency					C↑[e]	
Vitamin D					C↓[f]	C↓[g]
Vitamin E supplements			C-NR			
Folate			P↓			
Minerals						
High sodium intake			C↑			
Salt-preserved foods and salt				P↑[h]		
Potassium			C↓			
Calcium						C↓[g]
Fluoride, local					C↓[c]	
Fluoride, systemic					C↓[c]	P-NR[g]
Fluoride, excess					C↑[f]	
Hypocalcaemia					P↑[f]	
Meat and fish						
Preserved meat				P↑[i]		
Chinese-style salted fish				C↑[j]		

	Obesity	Type 2 diabetes	CVD	Cancer	Dental disease	Osteoporosis
Fruits (including berries) and vegetables						
Fruits (including berries) and vegetables	C↓[k]	P↓[k]	C↓	P↓[l]		
Whole fresh fruits					P-NR[c]	
Beverages, non-alcoholic						
Sugars-sweetened soft drinks and fruit juices	P↑				P↑[m]	
Very hot (thermally) drinks (and food)				P↑[n]		
Unfiltered boiled coffee			P↑			
Beverages, alcoholic						
High alcohol intake			C↑[o]	C↑[p]		C↑[g]
Low to moderate alcohol intake			C↓[q]			
Other food-borne						
Aflatoxins				C↑[r]		
Weight and physical activity						
Abdominal obesity		C↑				
Overweight and obesity		C↑	C↑	C↑[s]		
Voluntary weight loss in overweight and obese people		C↓				
Low body weight						C↑[g]
Physical activity, regular	C↓	C↓	C↓	C↓[i] P↓[t]		C↓[g]
Physical inactivity/sedentary lifestyle	C↑	C↑				
Other factors						
Exclusive breastfeeding	P↓					
Maternal diabetes		C↑				
Intrauterine growth retardation		P↑				
Good oral hygiene/absence of plaque					C↓[e]	
Hard cheese					P↓[c]	
Environmental variables						
Home and school environments that support healthy food choices for children	P↓					
Heavy marketing of energy-dense foods, and fast-food outlets	P↑					
Adverse socioeconomic conditions	P↑					

C↑: Convincing increasing risk; C↓: Convincing decreasing risk; C-NR: Convincing, no relationship; P↑: Probable increasing risk; P↓: Probable decreasing risk; P-NR: Probable, no relationship; EPA: eicosapentaenoic acid; DHA: docosahexaenoic acid; NSP: non-starch polysaccharides.

[a] Only convincing (C) and probable (P) evidence are included in this summary table.
[b] Evidence also summarized for selected specific fatty acids, see myristic and palmitic acid.
[c] For dental caries.
[d] Includes cooked and raw starch foods, such as rice, potatoes and bread. Excludes cakes, biscuits and snacks with added sugar.
[e] For periodontal disease.
[f] For enamel developmental defects.
[g] In populations with high fracture incidence only; applies to men and women more than 50–60 years old.
[h] For stomach cancer.
[i] For colorectal cancer.
[j] For nasopharyngeal cancer.
[k] Based on the contributions of fruits and vegetables to non-starch polysaccharides.
[l] For cancer of the oral cavity, oesophagus, stomach and colorectum.
[m] For dental erosion.
[n] For cancer of the oral cavity, pharynx and oesophagus.
[o] For stroke.
[p] For cancer of the oral cavity, pharynx, larynx, oesophagus, liver and breast.
[q] For coronary heart disease.
[r] For liver cancer.
[s] For cancer of the oesophagus, colorectum, breast (in postmenopausal women), endometrium and kidney.
[t] For breast cancer.